THE GOLDEN BOOK
OF MUSCLE HEALTH AND RESTORATION

by

MICHAEL R. BINDER, M.D.

THE UNIVERSITY OF CHICAGO, PRITZKER SCHOOL OF MEDICINE

AND

UCLA DEPARTMENT OF KINESIOLOGY

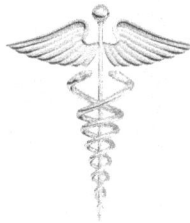

Note: the information in this book is for educational purposes and is not intended for use as a substitute for formal evaluation and treatment. Anyone with severe or persistent musculoskeletal pain or impairment should consult with a knowledgeable healthcare practitioner.

Author's Preface

I had been in perfect health with a thriving psychiatric practice until the age of forty-five when I suffered a sudden attack of kidney stones. Due to an unfortunate delay in diagnosis, I was laid up for several months before I was able to resume my normal activities. Shortly after returning to regular exercise, I tweaked something deep in my abdomen while doing squatting exercises. I wasn't sure what I had injured, but it felt like either a muscle deep in my hip or a disc in my lower back. Anyhow, I immediately discontinued the exercise and awoke the next morning feeling fine. But about a week later, I began to experience tiny electrical shocks around my right hip while jogging. I thought perhaps it was related to what had happened while doing squats, but since I had been feeling fine otherwise, I decided that I would just avoid jogging for the summer and swim instead.

However, in the weeks that followed, I started to notice other unusual things. I began to experience lower back pain and tightness down the side of my right thigh toward the end of a round of golf. I also began to experience an odd sensation along the side of my right foot and intermittent pain in my right hip that eventually progressed to the point of difficulty climbing stairs. The whole thing came to a head after I lifted a heavy table and developed continuous nerve pain down the back of my right thigh. On formal evaluation, a chiropractor diagnosed what I had feared: a spinal disc was bulging and irritating a nerve in my lower back. She recommended a course of message therapy and assured me that I would be all right.

Unfortunately, that's not how it turned out. On the contrary, I gradually got worse until I couldn't do anything; I couldn't jog, I couldn't play golf, I couldn't even clean my car because the nerve pain was prohibiting me from bending or even walking normally. So I scheduled an appointment with a prominent orthopedist at Northwestern University. After thoroughly examining me, he too thought that a bulging disc was causing my symptoms. He recommended physical therapy, which I began a few days later.

Unfortunately, the therapy was completely ineffective. In fact, some of the exercises made my symptoms worse. Although I considered returning to the orthopedist, I did not want to try anything invasive, so I went to see another chiropractor. Although this second chiropractor assured me that the "adjustments" and simple exercises she recommended could not possibly do me any harm, one of the exercises did. And so at my insistence, she ordered an MRI. The imaging study showed a mildly herniated disc at the L5-S1 interspace with a small left-central protrusion. The odd thing was that all my symptoms were on the right; my left leg was completely unaffected. And so began a four-year-long quest to figure out what was really wrong with me. Over those years, I consulted five primary care doctors, three orthopedic surgeons, twelve chiropractors, four physical therapists, five athletic trainers, three massage therapists, and spent over one hundred hours in physical therapy without any improvement or even an accurate diagnosis!

Then one night out of sheer desperation, I begged God to help me. It was the most passionate prayer I had ever said. The very next day, I learned of a unique treatment that was based on a highly precise and detailed understanding of neuromuscular physiology. Having a degree in Kinesiology, I was able to understand and appreciate the scientific, scholarly, and profound nature of the information presented. It was just what I had been looking for because until then, no one I consulted had been able to give me a clear anatomical or physiological explanation for my symptoms.

By God's providence, I was referred to Ms. Sharon Drewett, a practitioner of what is formally known as KANON myotherapy. The acronym "KANON" stands for Kinetically Activated Nerve Organ Normalization, which is the means by which the therapy had the potential to correct my problem.

In reviewing my original injury, Ms. Drewett reasoned that I had probably overloaded my right psoas muscle, creating an acute spasm that had become disabling because so much of the muscle had already been in a state that she called "hypertonic spasm." As you will learn, hypertonic spasm is an abnormal sustained contraction of muscle that silently develops over the course of many years as a result of sustained inactivity, or, in some cases, over-activity, and is permanent unless treated. As I thought about it, the whole thing made a lot of sense. As a psychiatrist, I spend almost all of my time sitting, which made me a prime candidate for hypertonic spasm. When I had returned to exercise after the kidney stone, I overloaded one of my already hypertonic muscles and was unable to recover because both the injured muscle and the surrounding muscles had so little healthy reserve. The discussion of this commonly misdiagnosed condition, its treatment, and its prevention are the subject of this book.

This book is written in honor of Sir Thomas Griner, a former research engineering technician at NASA who revolutionized the treatment of chronic musculoskeletal pain by identifying the most common cause of the problem and developing the only reliable way to cure it.

Through more than twenty-five years of research and clinical practice, Dr. Griner discovered the complex mechanism by which a seemingly simple yet intricate non-invasive bio-stimulation technique, one that he himself developed, could, over time, fully release hypertonic spasm, a dysfunctional state of muscle that is at the root of most cases of acute and chronic musculoskeletal pain.

Logical but revolutionary, simple but powerfully effective, Dr. Griner's discovery and the science behind it make him worthy of the Nobel Prize in physiology.

TABLE OF CONTENTS

What you are about to read is revolutionary. It is by far the most exciting scientific discovery that I have come across in twenty years as a physician. It is the hidden truth about the largest tissue in the body--muscle--and how it functions in sickness and in health.

Based on scientific facts and clinical success on the toughest cases in the fields of spinal medicine and physical rehabilitation, the information in this book is the beginning of a new era in the prevention and treatment of musculoskeletal pain and dysfunction. We're talking about preserving muscle health and vitality into old age and completely healing some of the most treatment-resistant cases of chronic musculoskeletal pain in a way that is sensible, scientific, and safe.

CHAPTER 1

OVERVIEW OF THE PROBLEM

This book is written for people of all ages from all walks of life. It is as much for the professional athlete as for the office secretary, as much for the young teen as for the aging grandparent. It is about a little known but extremely important factor in our health called *hypertonic muscle spasm*. All of us have it to some degree, but until it progresses to the point of pain, injury, or sickness, its insidious onset is either completely silent or perceived as nothing more than an inevitable age-related decline in flexibility and strength. We'll begin by discussing its relevance to those who suffer from chronic musculoskeletal pain and follow with its equal importance to those who are in good health and would like to optimize their fitness and longevity.

One quarter of the United States population suffers from chronic lower back pain, and fully half of the population suffers from some form of neck, shoulder, knee, hip, or temporomandibular joint (TMJ) pain. In addition to the emotional burden this places on the sufferers and their families, the financial burden is staggering. The annual loss of work productivity due to these conditions is estimated to be nearly fifty billion dollars, and the healthcare costs are exorbitant when you consider that the average pain patient consults multiple, sometimes even dozens of healthcare professionals in an effort to find relief.

The high prevalence and enormous toll of these conditions is largely due to a blind spot in the healthcare profession when it comes to musculoskeletal pain. The general assumption has been and continues to be that pain and other symptoms of nerve irritation are caused by a structural abnormality such as a herniated disc, arthritic joint, or torn cartilage that may be seen on an X-ray or MRI (magnetic resonance imaging). To be sure, there are cases where this is true, but far more often the structural abnormality, when present, has nothing to do with the symptoms. The increasing availability of MRI, though useful in many ways, has loaned itself to the misinterpretation of symptoms because imaging studies are able to detect structural abnormalities without sensitivity to their diagnostic significance1 or the length of time they have been present. Consequently, new-onset and chronic pain are often misattributed to abnormalities that are merely coincidental findings, often having been present for years, sometimes even decades before the symptoms began. Even more concerning is that invasive procedures such as steroid injections and surgery are often performed on these coincidental abnormalities, unnecessarily placing patients at risk for complications such as infection, nerve damage, and scarring, not to mention the emotional and financial burden it places on the patient, the family, and the medical system.

This leads to the question: if most pain is not caused by a structural abnormality, then what could be causing it? To answer that question, let us begin by discussing pain. Pain is a perception that is normally triggered by stimulation of sensory organs at the endings of a nerve. For example, if you prick your finger, nerve-endings in the skin initiate an electrical impulse that is conveyed along the length of the nerve, up the spinal cord, and into the brain, from where it is interpreted by the psyche. However, the same sensation could be produced by stimulating the nerve anywhere along its path. For example, if the nerve is irritated at the elbow, it could again feel as though someone is pricking your finger, and, oddly enough, this can occur without any sensation of pain at the elbow. Thus, the pain itself does not necessarily tell us the location of its source or what is causing it. The nature of the sensation can also vary, depending upon which nerve-endings or nerve fibers are being stimulated. Some fibers convey touch, others vibration, others pain and temperature.

What is so often overlooked in the assessment of pain is that nerves travel through and between muscles en route to their destinations and that muscles, because of their ability to create tension, can pinch, squeeze, and irritate nerves. Because the sensation of nerve irritation does not necessarily tell us the form or location of the irritation, a nerve can be irritated by a muscle in its path yet feel as though it is irritated by something else in its path. For example, the sensation of pain down the back of your leg could be caused by a spastic muscle in your hip; or tingling in your fingers could be caused by a spastic muscle in your neck. Hence, muscles can irritate nerves covertly, particularly because muscle tightness and spasm do not themselves necessarily cause pain or discomfort. To be sure, muscle tension can be palpated and the proper assessment made by a knowledgable practitioner, but the significance of hypertonic spasm is a relatively new discovery and still unknown to most clinicians. Another barrier to the diagnosis is that high-tech imaging studies have all but replaced the traditional physical examination, and these studies are more sensitive to structural abnormalities than to soft tissue abnormalities such as tight muscles. Consequently, abnormalities like a herniated disc, an arthritic joint, or a torn cartilage, which are visible on imaging studies, are often mistaken as the cause of symptoms that are actually due to spastic muscles.

One of the most commonly mistaken sights of nerve irritation is the point where nerves exit the spinal column. Sciatica and related musculoskeletal symptoms have historically been attributed to impingement of nerve roots as they exit the spine. This dogma is so entrenched that an entire medical specialty--the field of chiropractic--has been built around it, and orthopedists perform thousands of surgeries every year to correct associated abnormalities of the spine. However, recent studies have found little correlation between MRI pathology and either the patient's symptoms or course of improvement.[2,3] In March, 2013, a research team led by Wilco Peul, MD, PhD reported that at one year follow-up for disc surgery to treat sciatica, the majority of patients without any remaining symptoms had continued evidence of disc herniation.[3] The study, which was published in *The New England Journal of Medicine*, was conducted at nine centers and included 283 patients. When the patients were divided into two groups, eighty-five percent of those with continued evidence of disc herniation reported a favorable outcome, while eighty-three percent of those without continued evidence of disc herniation reported a favorable outcome. The study demonstrated that the presence of disc herniation at one year follow-up was unrelated to whether symptoms persisted or not. The researchers concluded that the lack of correlation between symptoms and MRI findings remains unclear. In an earlier study, researchers at UCLA and the Nerve Institute in Los Angeles reported that standard MRI imaging, though able to detect abnormalities of the spine, is unable to specify whether such abnormalities are irritating nerves. However, they did find that a new imaging technique called Magnetic Resonance Neurography can diagnose piriformis syndrome, a form of sciatica caused by "a narrow muscle deep in the pelvis." The researchers went on to say that "although sciatica is the most common condition treated by neurosurgeons, piriformis syndrome is not even mentioned in the majority of neurosurgery textbooks, and no more than a handful of surgeons in the United States are trained to treat it..." The authors concluded by saying: "For the last seventy years, sciatica has been thought to be caused by a herniated disc and treated as such. But our study shows that it is time for a major reassessment of how patients will be evaluated and treated for sciatica in the future..."[1]

This underscores the relevance of muscle in the assessment and treatment of musculoskeletal pain. The average person is two-thirds muscle, and that creates far more opportunity for nerve irritation than any of the common structural abnormalities when you consider that nerves weave through and between layers of overlapping muscles that have the ability to compress, pinch, and squeeze them.

Yet apart from its relationship to a few rare diseases, the relevance of muscle is largely overlooked by the medical profession. I attended two prominent medical schools in the United States and was taught little about muscle structure and function and its relevance to chronic pain and other medical conditions. Perhaps because of its natural association with strength and physical performance, muscle is rarely thought of as a vast supportive tissue of blood vessels, nerves, and lymphatics, whose function can markedly affect our health. Today, there is a medical subspecialty for every organ and tissue of the body, yet there remains none for muscle. There are still no "myologists" in the ever-expanding field of medicine, though we are covered with muscle from head to toe.

The relevance of muscle is that it can interfere with bodily functions as readily as it can support them. The essential role of skeletal muscle, which is the kind of muscle to which we are referring, is to maintain the structure of the body while allowing it to move with strength, precision,

(a)

(b)

Deep Femoral Artery
and Vein

Rectus Femoris Muscle

Sartorius Muscle

Vastus Intermedius
Muscle

Femoral Vein
and Artery

Femur Bone

Abbductor
Longus Muscle

Vastus Lateralis
Muscle

Gracilis
Muscle

Perforating
Artery and Vein

Schiatic
Nerve

Biceps Femoris Muscle

Semimembranosus
Muscle

Semitendinosus
Muscle

Schiatic
Nerve

Biceps Femoris
Muscle

Tibial
Nerve

Common
Peroneal
Nerve

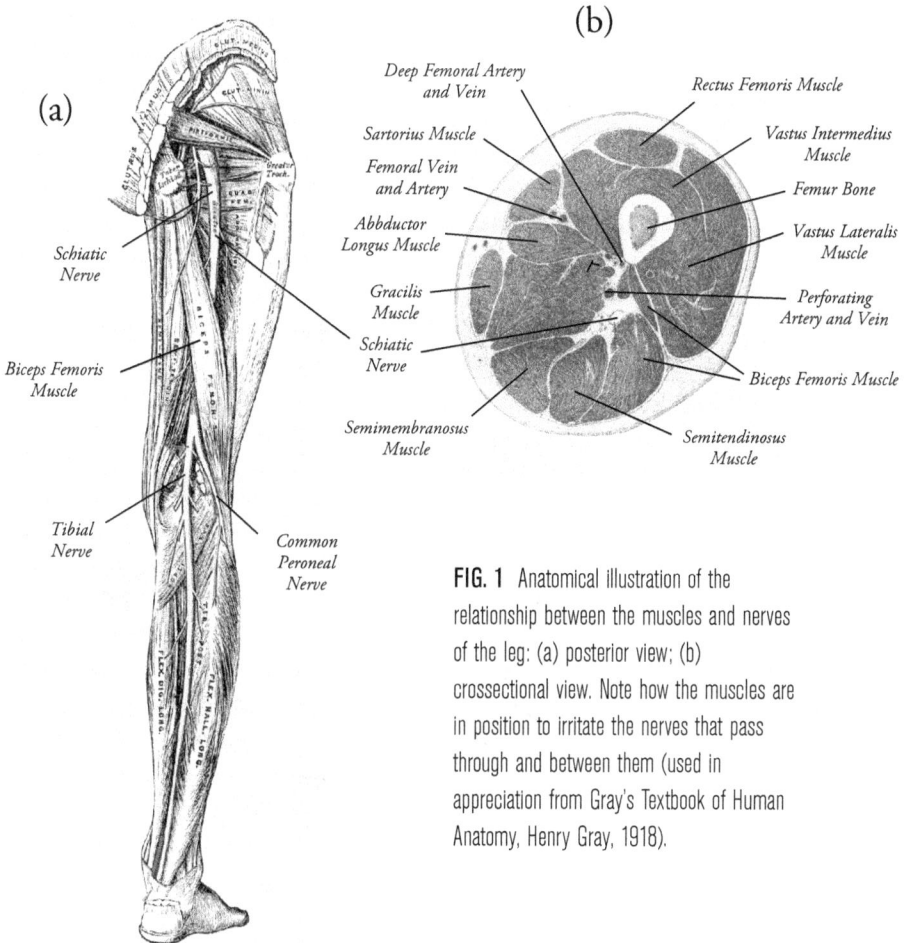

FIG. 1 Anatomical illustration of the relationship between the muscles and nerves of the leg: (a) posterior view; (b) crossectional view. Note how the muscles are in position to irritate the nerves that pass through and between them (used in appreciation from Gray's Textbook of Human Anatomy, Henry Gray, 1918).

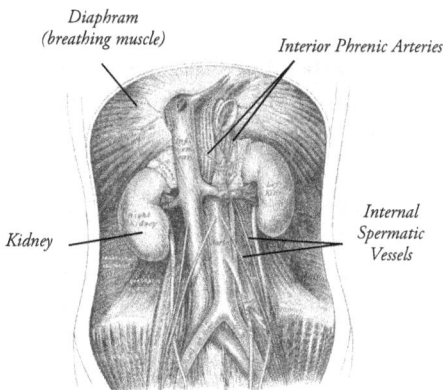

Diaphram
(breathing muscle)

Interior Phrenic Arteries

Internal
Spermatic
Vessels

Kidney

FIG. 2 Illustration of the anatomical interface between skeletal muscles and various organs and tissues of the body (used in appreciation from Gray's Textbook of Human Anatomy, Henry Gray, 1918).

and ease. To accomplish this, skeletal muscle is under both conscious and unconscious control. This is in contrast to smooth muscle and cardiac muscle, which are exclusively under unconscious control. Skeletal muscles are attached to every bone in the body and support every joint to provide an adaptable structural framework for all of our organs and tissues. Therefore, when skeletal muscles are healthy, they provide structure and support for the heart, lungs, kidneys, and other organs, as well as for the blood vessels, lymphatics, and nerves that serve those organs. But if the muscles become unhealthy, all the organs and tissues of the body can be adversely affected because all of them interface with skeletal muscles either directly or indirectly.

Physical therapists and athletic trainers are well-versed in addressing the problem of weak muscles, but few are versed in the problem of sick muscles. Perhaps some of us have heard of fibromyalgia or rare neuromuscular diseases like muscular dystrophy and myasthenia gravis, but who has heard of the far more common and highly relevant phenomenon of hypertonic muscle spasm? Hypertonic spasm is an abnormal, sustained contraction of skeletal muscle that impairs muscle function and creates a hostile environment for local nerves, organs, and tissues, including other muscles, and is actually the most common cause of acute and chronic musculoskeletal pain and dysfunction.

When I was suffering from sciatica (symptoms associated with irritation of the sciatic nerve), I consulted more than twenty medical specialists, and only one of them conceptualized muscle spasm as the root of the problem. Unfortunately, he was unable to help me due to a lack of sufficient knowledge in the area of muscle. To be sure, the relevance of muscle in both sickness and health continues to go largely unrecognized, as does its proper treatment. Consequently, an alarmingly high percentage of patients who suffer from chronic muscle spasm are being misdiagnosed and mismanaged. To change this, we need to start addressing the problem of hypertonic spasm.

+ + +

CHAPTER 2

PHYSIOETIOLOGY OF HYPERTONIC SPASM

In order to understand how skeletal muscles become hypertonic, let us first review the structure and function of healthy muscle. Skeletal muscle is comprised of cylindrically-shaped cells called *muscle fibers* that contain highly organized rows of contractile filaments called *actin* and *myosin*. What causes a muscle to contract is the passage of these filaments past one another through an action akin to rowing a boat. The oars on the filaments are powered by the oxidative breakdown of a chemical called *adenosine triphosphate (ATP)* in conjunction with the sudden release of calcium from storage compartments within the muscle cells in response to a nerve signal from the brain.

The majority of the muscle cells or "fibers" within a muscle have only one job: to contract. But scattered throughout the muscle are smaller, spindle-shaped contractile units called *muscle spindles* that continuously monitor the length, the change of length, the rate of change of length, and the tension in the muscle. Continuous feedback from muscle spindles is what allows us to maintain our position in space and perform complex movements with ease and precision.

It was once believed that a resting muscle had zero tension. But what has become clear from studying denervated muscle in comparison to healthy muscle is that there is always a minimal amount of tension in resting healthy muscle that is calibrated by the cerebellum of the brain. The cerebellum monitors this tension via constant feedback from the muscle spindles. However, a breakdown product of muscle metabolism called *lactic acid* can interfere with the spindle's feedback to the cerebellum.

Under most conditions, interference with spindle feedback does not occur because the products of muscle metabolism are whisked away by the circulatory system before they can back up into the muscle spindles. However, if circulation fails to keep up with lactic acid production, lactic acid can begin to accumulate and seep into the muscle spindles. When this occurs, feedback from the muscle spindles to the cerebellum about the resting tension of the muscle becomes blunted. The cerebellum interprets the blunted feedback as an indication that the muscle is too loose, so it orders up more tension. The increased tension ramps up the accumulation of lactic acid both because it increases the rate at which the metabolite is produced and because the muscle contraction itself cuts off circulation, thus trapping more lactic acid in the muscle. The rising concentration of lactic acid further blunts feedback to the cerebellum, causing it to order up even more tension in the muscle. Eventually, the muscle can become so tight that even at rest the rate of lactic acid production begins to exceed the rate at which it can be removed, resulting in a sustained, self-perpetuating contraction called *hypertonic spasm*. The accumulation of lactic acid within a hypertonic muscle not only keeps the muscle in spasm, but it can gradually diffuse into neighboring muscles and eventually lead them into spasm. In a sense, muscles have all the ingredients to make cement, and if we do not flush them out on a regular basis through movement and healthy exercise, the cement will begin to harden. Hardened muscle is dysfunctional because muscles must relax and contract in order to function normally.

Whenever skeletal muscles contract, core fibers are recruited first. Hence, when hypertonic spasm develops, it begins in the core of the muscle and grows outward. An expanding core of spastic muscle can take decades to develop to the point where it becomes noticeable to the individual. Until then, it grows asymptomatically as long as there are enough non-spastic fibers remaining in the more superficial layers of the muscle to meet the demands placed upon them. But if the body is asked to do something that overwhelms the muscles, such as a heavy lift, a prolonged activity, or an awkward movement, the muscles can go into acute spasm. Spastic muscles are stiff and can irritate local nerves, causing pain, numbness, tingling, and other symptoms of nerve irritation. The muscle spasm can be self-sustaining because the lactic acid that it traps causes the muscle to remain contracted. It's like grabbing a live wire; when you feel the electricity, you want to let go but you can't because the electricity is causing the muscles of your hand to remain contracted. This can be excruciatingly painful! Acute pain of this sort is a leading cause of visits to the emergency room and the primary care doctor.

Now then, because the medical profession has a blind spot when it comes to muscle, the ubiquitous phenomenon of hypertonic spasm is rarely considered, and the search for the source of musculoskeletal pain is typically limited to the skeletal system. So if the pain is in your back, you can expect an X-ray or MRI of your back. If the pain is in your neck, you can expect the same tests of your neck. The same work-up is done for pain in the shoulder, hip, knee, and any other part of the skeletal system. When the imaging studies show a structural abnormality such as a herniated disc, an arthritic joint, or a torn cartilage, what is seen on film is assumed to be the cause of the symptoms. Rarely is any consideration given to the possibility that the pain and other symptoms could be stemming from the neuromuscular system. Even when prior imaging studies document that the structural abnormality had been present long before the symptoms began, the assumption remains the same. Somewhat illogically, it is assumed that the abnormality was not causing symptoms then but is now. Hence, treatment is typically aimed at what is seen on film. So if there is a herniated disc, one might be given a spinal injection; if there is an arthritic knee, one might be prescribed an anti-inflammatory drug; if there is a torn cartilage, surgery; if there is an injured rotator cuff, physical therapy. Because physical therapy is non-invasive and has been found to be helpful for many patients with the aforementioned conditions, it is usually recommended as a safe, first-line therapy. The general assumption is that strengthening muscles around a structural abnormality can alleviate symptoms by "stabilizing the joint." But in most cases, the muscles are already too tight because they are in spasm. In fact, it is this excess tension that tends to cause discs to bulge and joints to become arthritic! Yet strengthening muscles through physical therapy can help. The means by which physical therapy can reduce symptoms of nerve irritation involves two distinct but interrelated mechanisms. If begun soon enough after the onset of symptoms and performed in the right manner and at the right intensity, loosening and strengthening can help flush enough of the accumulated lactic acid out of the superficial layers of spastic muscle to partially relax the tissue. As the muscles begin to relax, nerve irritation is reduced, and symptoms begin to resolve. Over time, physical therapy can also strengthen large groups of muscles, which reduces the load on any given muscle, thereby reducing the risk of re-injury. However, excessive exercise can cause lactic acid to be produced faster than it can be flushed out, and improper exercise can cause spastic muscles to tighten even further through a protective mechanism called the *stretch reflex*. Both processes can result in the further accumulation of lactic acid, causing the already spastic muscles to become even more spastic and symptoms to become more severe. That's why physical therapy is helpful for some but not for others and in some cases can even makes things worse. Even when physical therapy is effective, the spastic muscles are only partially reconditioned; the core of hypertonicity remains, leaving the patient continually at risk for a recurrence of symptoms. Hence the saying, "once you have a bad back, you always have a bad back," and "once you injure a shoulder or knee, it's never quite the same."

+ + +

CHAPTER 3

WHAT WE DO (OR DON'T DO) THAT CAUSES OUR MUSCLES TO BECOME HYPERTONIC

B ased on the physioetiology of hypertonic spasm, we know that anything that causes lactic acid to accumulate in a muscle sets the stage for the development of hypertonus. There are three fundamental ways that lactic acid can accumulate in skeletal muscles: underuse, overuse, and improper use.

As previously discussed, muscles maintain some degree of tension or "tone" even at rest. In maintaining that tension, a small amount of lactic acid is continually produced. This lactic acid cannot be adequately eliminated without enough physical activity on a regular basis to permit healthy circulation.

The problem of underuse actually begins in the womb. By the fifth month of gestation, the muscular system of the fetus has already formed, but because there is so little room for movement, the "round" muscles of the body begin to accumulate lactic acid. The round muscles are those like the biceps (in the arms) and the hamstrings (in the legs) that, for functional purposes, are arranged in concentric circles. While this arrangement is a functional necessity, it cuts off circulation when the muscles contract, thus allowing lactic acid to accumulate and poison the muscle spindles. The tightly contracted arms and legs of a screaming newborn are evidence of this. The spastic limb contraction is not so much caused by the stress of the birth process as it is by the constricted quarters of the womb. Although the freedom of movement enjoyed after birth allows most of the accumulated lactic acid to be flushed out of the muscles, a small amount remains permanently trapped deep in the core of the muscle. The good news is that our muscles have plenty of reserve capacity, which is why this deep core of hypertonus is functionally insignificant. However, if we don't move our muscles on a regular basis, lactic acid will begin to re-accumulate in the remaining healthy muscle tissue. That's the primary reason that prolonged sitting is so unhealthy, particularly for the weight-bearing lower body. The stiffness you feel after sitting for a long time tells you that the muscles are becoming poisoned with lactic acid. As you begin to walk around, circulation returns to the affected muscles, and the accumulated lactic acid begins to diffuse out of the spindles, allowing the muscles to loosen up. But unless prolonged sedentariness is balanced with healthy exercise to thoroughly flush out and rejuvenate the muscles, they will eventually become permanently poisoned, which is the state called hypertonic spasm.

The second fundamental way that skeletal muscles can accumulate lactic acid and, thus, become hypertonic is through overuse. Overuse activities are those that strain muscles continually. The continuous strain causes lactic acid to accumulate by choking off circulation for an extended period of time. An example would be prolonged holding of the telephone trapped between the ear and shoulder. The continuous strain tends to cause lactic acid to accumulate in the muscles of the neck and shoulder. Another example would be housecleaning in positions where the head is continually held unsupported, such as when cleaning bathtubs, floors, or baseboards. This places continuous strain on the muscles of the neck, often resulting in pain and stiffness. Another potentially compromising activity is house-painting because it typically involves holding the brush or roller with the arm extended for prolonged periods. Note that the common element in these examples is a prolonged, isometric-type contraction that prevents the circulatory system from flushing lactic acid out of the tissue. The problem could be avoided by allowing short but frequent periods of rest.

A third way to develop hypertonic spasm is through improper exercise. Any exercise that involves a strenuous muscle contraction for more than about five to six seconds without a relaxation phase will produce more lactic acid in the working round muscles than can be removed by the restricted circulation. Common examples are prolonged holding of a bridge pose or performing too many repetitions in exercises such as pushups and squats. Over time, these unhealthy exercise routines can cause the resting tension in the muscles to increase, just as occurs with prolonged sedentariness. The veins of a bodybuilder pop to the surface because the deeper veins are choked off by hard, permanently contracted muscle. Over time, this lack of venous circulation can cause the affected muscles to develop an ever-expanding core of hypertonicity that can grow to the point where all that remains is a thin layer of functional muscle, thus making an individual increasingly susceptible to pain, spasm, and injury. Although this does not strictly apply to flat muscles like the latissimus dorsi, even the flat muscles are susceptible because of the tendency for lactic acid to become trapped where the tendon cups into its boney attachment. Most bodybuilders are walking around with tight, chronically contracted muscles because they routinely violate the six-second rule in their exercise routines. Unlike powerlifters, who lift weight for just a few seconds before putting it down, bodybuilders continue to pump the weight without a break, which has the effect of restricting blood flow through the working muscles to the point where the contraction or "pump" is partially retained even at rest. Although this might look attractive, it has several unhealthy effects. First, the chronic contraction reduces flexibility, which tends to cause one to become "musclebound." Second, inflexible muscles are prone to spasm, which is what occurs when you "throw out your back." Third, chronic muscle tension places a continuous strain on joints and tendons that over time can lead to vertebral disc herniations, painful calcifications, arthritis, and other complications. Fourth, blood vessels and nerves that pass through and between spastic muscles are constantly compressed and irritated, which reduces blood flow and neurological input to the organs and tissues they serve. This can lead to or accentuate a number of general health problems including high blood pressure, migraine headaches, chronic fatigue, depression, asthma, allergies, herpes, and a range of metabolic and rheumatologic disorders.

Underuse, overuse, and improper exercise are not the only ways to develop hypertonic spasm. Anything that offsets the balance between lactic acid production and removal can potentially lead to hypertonic spasm. That can include a wide range of common activities from lifting something that is too heavy to a simple bend or twist. Even emotional stress can contribute because nervous tension causes muscles to tighten and blood vessels to constrict, both of which upset the circulatory balance. The most susceptible are the illiopsoas and lower back muscles (involved in sitting, standing, and walking) because they tend to have a large burden of hypertonicity as a result of prolonged subjection to the three fundamental causes of hypertonic spasm--overuse, underuse, and improper exercise.

The lag time between an episode of acute spasm and the development of hypertonic spasm explains why some injuries, such as a whiplash or a fall can produce immediate symptoms (the acute spasm) that seem to completely resolve only to reemerge months or even years later. It's as if the affected muscles retain a memory of the injury that makes them more susceptible to re-injury and the reemergence of symptoms. Their "memory" represents the development of hypertonic spasm.

One of the things that makes the development of hypertonic spasm so sneaky is that there are few if any symptoms until the compromised muscles reach their tipping point. The tipping point is where the daily demands on the muscle exceed the reserve capacity of the remaining healthy fibers. At that point, the superficial fibers of the muscle, which are always the last to become hypertonic, start to become overwhelmed with increasing frequency, causing more and more of them to become like the hypertonic core. This not only places a greater burden on synergist (helper) muscles, but it can also lead them into hypertonic spasm by one or a combination of four mechanisms. A spastic muscle can lead neighboring muscles into spasm by directly irritating them; by leaking lactic acid into them; by reducing circulation to them; and by irritating nerves that reflex to them. As more and more muscle tissue becomes hypertonic, the cascade becomes a slippery slope with an accelerating loss of functional capacity. To the sufferer, pain becomes more frequent and severe as nerves become irritated more often and with the simplest movements. This in turn increases the frequency of reflex spasm and the severity of the other components in the cascade. In an effort to guard against the progression of symptoms, the individual is forced to become increasingly cautious by moving slower and doing less.

By now you know that restricting activity feeds right into the problem because it further reduces circulation to the muscles.

Through my own hellish experience, I understand this process from its inconspicuous beginning to its crippling end. I had for more than a decade had hypertonic spasm in muscles around my right hip joint. Yet I had no symptoms except for a soft creaking that I could both hear and feel while I was doing range-of-motion exercises. Although the crepitus made me wonder whether I was developing arthritis in the hip, there was no pain, weakness, or restriction of movement, so I just dismissed it.

Then, in 2008, I tweaked a muscle deep in that same hip while doing squats. It was the same muscle I had strained years earlier while doing seated rows at the gym. Much like the previous episode, the pain was a momentary twinge, just severe enough to convince me to discontinue the exercise. There were no persistent symptoms, and when I got out of bed the next morning, I felt fine. But during the following weeks, I began to experience mild intermittent shocks around my right hip while jogging. I also began to have stiffness in the hip after prolonged sitting or walking. By the end of that summer, I could barely climb a flight of stairs because the strain on the hip made it feel as though it were broken. I also began to experience intermittent pain in my lower back and increased sensitivity to touch along the side of my right foot. What I would eventually discover was that the squatting exercise had thrown a muscle that was already hypertonic deeper into spasm.

In retrospect, the warning signs of hypertonic spasm were the longstanding crepitus in the hip and the repeated injuries in the area with a progression of symptoms to local pain and the paraesthesia in my right foot. As previously discussed, hypertonic spasm begins in the core of round muscles and extends outward over time, irritating local nerves, impacting neighboring muscles, and gradually reducing the functional capacity of the muscle as a whole. This in turn leaves the remaining healthy fibers of the muscle increasingly vulnerable to acute spasm and eventual incorporation into the growing core of hypertonicity.

The whole thing came to a head after I lifted a heavy table and held it in a locked, standing position. I did not experience any symptoms of injury at the time, but the next morning I noticed an unusual tightness in my right thigh and a return of numbness in my right foot. A few days later, I began to experience pain radiating down the back of my thigh.

Why the delay in onset of symptoms? Because spastic muscle has to get tight enough and irritate local nerves enough to perceive that there is a problem. Still unaware of the cause of my symptoms, I felt certain that I had injured a nerve or herniated a disc in my lower back.

On formal evaluation by both a chiropractor and an orthopedic surgeon, I was diagnosed with a bulging disc. X-rays and an MRI of my right hip did not show any abnormalities, thus supporting the contention that the long-standing creaking in the hip was not caused by arthritis or a structural abnormality but by spastic muscle. An MRI of my lower back showed that I actually had a *herniated* disc at the L5-S1 interspace. However, the disc was protruding to the side opposite my symptoms. Thus, I was having symptoms where I should not have been, and no symptoms where I should have been. Though the doctors could not explain the discrepancy, they accepted the herniated disc as the cause of my symptoms and tailored my treatment accordingly.

Unfortunately, none of the treatments were effective. In fact some of them made my symptoms worse. Others provided some benefit initially only to be undone after weeks or months of treatment. In some cases, one therapist or doctor told me to do just the opposite of what the other told me to do. Meanwhile, my overall functional capacity gradually declined despite no evidence of structural change on several subsequent MRI scans.

The degree of impairment that my condition developed into is worth noting. Over a period of three years, I went from a full range of normal activities to the point where I was unable to bend very far, unable to sit very long, and unable to stand for more than a few minutes. Eventually, I needed one and then two canes to walk. Although I was able to sleep comfortably, any spontaneous movements in bed carried the risk of irritating nerves and sending the associated muscles into acute spasm. Such occurrences became increasingly frequent as my condition deteriorated and more and more muscle went into hypertonic spasm. Each time a local nerve was irritated by a spastic muscle, I would experience a momentary electrical shock that would cause me to cry out in pain. Yet the problem was not so much the momentary pain as it was the profound debilitating effect that the nerve irritation had on local muscles. Each time a nerve was irritated, all the muscles in the region would tighten up, which in turn heightened the risk of further nerve irritation until the acute spasm had time to dissipate--typically days to weeks. In an effort to reduce the risk of further injury, I had to continuously monitor the rate and extent of every move I made and avoid any activities that could cause my muscles to further tighten and in turn further irritate local nerves. For more than a year, my condition was so bad that I could not even bear my own weight without driving my leg muscles deeper into spasm. That's why I needed two canes to walk and had to lean on something to offset the weight of even the lightest things I needed to carry. I was unable to perform any exercises except for swimming, and even in the water, I had to avoid any sudden, forceful, or jerky movements. Getting in and out of the pool was itself a problem, and at one point, I actually asked to use a poolside chair-lift. The entire downhill course was set off by a subtle tweak (acute spasm) of a single muscle--my right psoas--that was not identified and properly managed before more and more of the surrounding musculature had gone into hypertonic spasm. All I kept thinking while I was in treatment was what I had been told: that I had a herniated disc, which was a chronic condition.

All of the clinicians I saw viewed the problem the same way, with the exception of a few. But even those who did not think my symptoms were caused by the herniated disc were unable to help me. In all, I was evaluated by some thirty clinicians, all of whom seemed to be just as naive to the phenomenon of hypertonic spasm as I was. The lack of awareness of the problem by the medical and therapeutic community is the second factor that makes hypertonic spasm so invisible and so dangerous. And it's one of the reasons that this and other books on the topic are so needed.

The third factor that makes hypertonic spasm so invisible is the dogmatic view that structural abnormalities and the high-tech imaging studies that detect them explain musculoskeletal pain syndromes. The very fact that we can see a structural abnormality makes it easier to accept as an explanation for symptoms than something we cannot see. That is not to say that hypertonic spasm is invisible. Far from it; it is actually more visible than the structural abnormalities that require X-rays and expensive scans to see. The problem is that when we see it, we all too often don't know what we're looking at. Recall that the growing core of hypertonic spasm is actually the muscle crimping down and wringing itself out like a sponge. Over time, the tissue loses fluid, causing the muscle to shrink and appear smaller than it would were it in a healthy contraction. So the assumption is that the muscle has undergone atrophy, presumably as a result of nerve damage and decreased use. But the muscle is actually tight, not flaccid; it is drained of fluid, not necessarily strength because it is not suffering from disuse as much as overuse! The proper term for it is hypotrophy, not atrophy. And the condition is quite visible; it's just misidentified. It is also quite palpable to the few clinicians who know how to diagnose and treat it.

The fourth factor that makes hypertonic spasm so deceptive is that the patient does not necessarily feel as though the muscles are in spasm, nor does the nerve irritation feel as though it is due to muscle spasm. Instead, it feels like the nerve is being irritated by a herniated disc or some other structural abnormality such as an arthritic joint or torn cartilage. If there is a sense of muscle weakness, it is not due to nerve damage but to reluctance in the muscle caused by nerve irritation. Reluctance is the body's way of protecting itself from injury when pain is perceived. What's more, hypertonic muscles do not have the flexibility that is required to generate functional force. So attempting to use them will merely increase the spasm and likely also the pain. Another misleading phenomenon can be the presence of crepitus, a creaking noise that sounds and feels as though it is coming from an associated joint. In reality, it is the sound of tight muscles and tendons snapping past one another and adjacent tissues during movement. It's akin to the sound you hear when you snap your fingers, if you can imagine snapping them about five times per second under ear your skin. The muffled snapping is easily mistaken for arthritis or joint damage, especially if there is radiographic evidence of these abnormalities. When joint abnormalities are present, they are almost always secondary rather than primary--the result of the chronic stress placed on them by the spastic muscles that cross and support them.

Thus, hypertonic spasm typically progresses unchecked and misdiagnosed, engulfing more and more muscle tissue and reducing its reserve capacity until its victim finds him or her self trapped in a downhill spiral that has but one reliable remedy.

And what is that remedy?

18

The answer is simple but the science behind it is complex, which is one of the reasons that the definitive treatment has evaded us for so long. As previously discussed, hypertonus develops in layers, starting at the core of the muscle and growing outward as more and more of the muscle becomes locked in spasm. These are not layers of individual muscle fibers as much as they are layers of spastic trauma, each having engulfed whatever portion of the muscle that became locked in spasm during the associated phase of progression. As each new layer of hypertonicity formed, the frozen core of the muscle grew and replaced some of the healthier surface tissue, leaving less and less functional muscle.

Recall that what keeps the core of the muscle "frozen" is the fact that the feedback loop between the muscle and the brain (which normally regulates a healthy degree of muscle tone) is poisoned by lactic acid, a product of muscle contraction that is both trapped in the muscle by the spasm and excessively produced because of the spasm. Also recall that it is the spasm that causes the pain and other symptoms as the spastic muscles crimp down on and irritate the nerves that pass through and between them. So in order to relieve the symptoms, we have to relieve the spasm; and in order to relieve the spasm, we have to help the muscle rid itself of the lactic acid that is keeping it in spasm.

The problem is that the spasm is guarded by the stretch reflex, which is a neuromuscular feedback loop between stretch receptors in the muscle and motor neurons in the spinal cord that stimulates the muscle to contract whenever it is stretched too far or too quickly. The stretch reflex is what causes the knee-jerk response when the doctor stretches the patellar tendon by taping your knee with a reflex hammer. Recall that hypertonic spasm is maintained by the cerebellum of the brain, which unconsciously keeps the muscle too tight because trapped lactic acid interferes with the muscle's ability to tell the brain that it is maintaining more than enough resting tone. The trapped lactic acid also heightens the sensitivity of the stretch reflex so that relatively small perturbations of the muscle can trigger further spasm, and with it the further production and accumulation of lactic acid. This makes hypertonic muscle highly resistant to treatment. If efforts to forcibly loosen the muscle by massaging it, digging into it, pounding on it, or rolling it seem to be effective, it is NOT because the underlying problem has been corrected. On the contrary; it is because reflex spasm

19

has caused fast-twitch fibers to fatigue. When those fibers recover, the muscle is apt to become even more tight. The application of various forms of current or ultrasound will tend to have the same effect. Moderate cooling reduces circulation through muscle, and moderate heating increases circulation though to a lesser extent when muscles are hypertonic because of the mechanical resistance to blood flow. Extremes of temperature, such as icing and hot baths, cause thermal shock, which causes muscles to tighten. If either modality seems to help, it is because the stress on the body stimulates the production of endorphins (natural pain-killers) and because temperature extremes have an analgesic (pain-relieving) effect on nerve-endings. However, these effects are temporary and misleading because they do nothing to release the underlying spasm. As for exercise, neither stretching, strengthening, walking, or even swimming can release hypertonic spasm. I swam daily for over four years and made a conscientious effort to carefully loosen my muscles each day without one bit of improvement regardless of the technique I used. Then again, what proper exercise *can* do is prevent more muscle from becoming hypertonic.

In order to release hypertonic spasm, we must stimulate the muscle in such a way that we override the blunting effect that the trapped lactic acid has on the cerebellar feedback nerves without stimulating the stretch reflex. This would stimulate the cerebellum to reduce the resting tension in the muscle, thus reducing the production of lactic acid and allowing the accumulated lactic acid to be flushed out by the increased circulation permitted by a more relaxed muscle. That is precisely what KANON non-invasive stimulation does.

+ + +

CHAPTER 4

BACKGROUND OF A BRILLIANT DISCOVERY

Having studied muscle physiology at a university that at the time was touted to be a leader in the field, I am surprised that I had been taught so little about muscle spasm. But in looking back, the integrative work on how muscles develop chronic spasticity had not yet been published. It was during my college years that Dr. Thomas Griner, a chiropractic student and former research engineering technician at NASA, was hard at work in this area. In his efforts to develop a comprehensive understanding of muscle structure and function as it pertains to muscle spasm, Dr. Griner had enrolled in the California School of Chiropractic while independently studying the complex anatomy and physiology of muscle. His years of research and clinical practice culminated in a scientifically-based method of relieving chronically spastic muscle. The non-invasive technique involves gently stimulating nerve organs in the muscle to recalibrate the muscle's resting tension. What Dr. Griner called Kinetically Activated Nerve Organ Normalization (abbreviated "KANON") has become the only known reliable way to relieve chronically spastic muscle.

The goal of this precise, physiologically-based stimulatory technique is to break the cycle of spasm by allowing the cerebellum to properly reset the resting tension of the muscle being treated. To accomplish this, the flower-spray nerves of the muscle spindle cells, which keep the cerebellum apprised of the resting tension of the muscle, are manually stimulated in a way that avoids activating the annulospiral nerves, which trigger the unwanted stretch reflex. In so doing, the dampening effect that lactic acid has on the flower-spray nerves is overcome mechanically, thus giving the cerebellum the neurological feedback it needs to reduce the resting tension of the muscle. As the muscle relaxes, the production of lactic acid declines and circulation improves, thus facilitating the removal of the accumulated lactic acid and allowing the flower-spray nerves to resume normal function. With the resumption of healthy communication between the muscle and the brain, the resting tension and associated functions of the muscle return to normal. As long as a healthy balance of rest and exercise is subsequently maintained, the resting tension of the muscle will remain healthy. Thus, the health of sickened muscles can be completely restored, but in order to maintain that health, one must avoid the things that caused those muscles to become hypertonic in the first place.

As a complement to the fingertip stimulation, Dr. Griner engineered the development of the BioPulser®, a hand-held machine about the size of an iron with a pulsating head that, like the massage technique, is designed to mechanically overcome the dampening effect that lactic acid has on the flower-spray nerves. The instrument gently taps the muscle at a speed and vibrational frequency that avoids the stretch reflex as it stimulates corrective feedback to the cerebellum. Technically, the tapping too can be done by hand, but the percussion must be performed in an exact manor in order to avoid triggering the stretch reflex. The BioPulser® makes it a lot easier and is more precise.

Over the past few decades, the success of KANON non-invasive stimulation has led to a major breakthrough in our understanding of chronic musculoskeletal pain syndromes. The new-found ability to effectively treat chronic musculoskeletal pain by releasing spastic muscle has demonstrated that the problem is typically the reverse of what was thought: the problem actually begins with muscle, and the associated structural abnormality, when present, is either coincidental or caused by the muscle spasm itself. We're not talking about bone fractures, ligament tears, and other severe traumatic injuries in which muscle spasm is naturally reactive. Rather, we're talking about symptoms that persist even after a structural abnormality has undergone significant healing or that develop in the absence of any trauma. For example, if a skier were to slam into a tree and suffer a hip fracture, reactive spasm of muscles around the hip joint would be a normal protective response. But what about pain and spasm that persist even after the fracture has substantially healed? That's the kind of thing we're talking about. Or take the golfer with a bad knee who continues to have pain even after "successful" surgery. The hidden problem is hypertonic muscle spasm; the structural abnormality was likely either coincidental or secondary. As another example, consider the office secretary who bends to pick up a pencil and throws out her back. Clearly, the act of bending is not a traumatic injury, yet she might find herself in so much pain that she cannot straighten up. The root cause of the problem is almost certainly hypertonic spasm regardless of how bad her spine might look on MRI. When she bended over, tight, spastic muscles in her back irritated local nerves, causing pain and the guarding reflex. The guarding reflex is one of several mechanisms by which the nervous system tries to prevent further movement when a nerve is irritated.

Through the success of Dr. Griner and others who skillfully practice the limited pressure massage and BioPulser® techniques, it has become increasingly clear that the persistence of symptoms such as radiating pain, numbness, and tingling, which had long been thought to be due to structural abnormalities of the spine or joints, are frequently if not always due to chronic muscle spasm. This has dramatic and far-reaching implications for treatment. It also explains why physical therapy, which focuses on muscle, is so commonly recommended (though misunderstood) and why surgery, which targets structural abnormalities, is so often unsuccessful. To date, numerous chronic pain-suffers have been saved from addictive pain medications, risky injections, and dangerous surgeries because they came across this information in time to get safe and effective treatment.

+ + +

CHAPTER 5

TREATMENT

For the few clinicians who know how to restore the health of hypertonic muscle, there is no mystery behind alleviating chronic musculoskeletal pain; it is purely a matter of releasing the contracted muscle that is causing the pain. As already discussed, any abnormalities seen on imaging studies of the spine, whether they be a herniated disc, a spinal stenosis, an arthritic joint, or some other structural abnormality are, in most cases, irrelevant because muscle spasm is the beginning and end of the problem. The spine has little to do with it. However, tightly contracted spinal muscles can cause discs to bulge and nerve outlets to narrow. Over time, discs can herniate, joints can become arthritic, and other abnormalities can develop in the chronically stressed skeletal system. Because these structural abnormalities are not the cause of the problem but the consequence, any attempt to relieve symptoms by treating them is both misguided and potentially dangerous. Treatment should begin by targeting the root of the problem--spastic muscle.

The same could be said for most of the other areas of chronic musculoskeletal pain, including but not limited to neck pain, shoulder pain, hip pain, knee pain, ankle pain, foot pain, TMJ pain, and carpel tunnel. All too often, needless surgeries and other invasive procedures are performed for a "torn rotator cuff," a cracked knee meniscus, an arthritic joint, or a painful hand. That is not to say that the structural abnormalities seen on X-rays and MRIs are not present; it's just that they are rarely, if ever, the source of the pain. Symptoms such as numbness and tingling in a hand or foot, pain radiating down the arm or back of the leg, and burning in the groin or calf are caused by nerve irritation in areas where tight, spastic muscles are rubbing against and squeezing nerves like a vise. The muscle spasm also reduces strength and flexibility, both of which lead to increased muscle spasticity by reducing movement. So if you're in pain and having trouble moving, it is most likely due to tight muscles, and something needs to be done to relieve the spasm. The skeleton of the body is just an innocent bystander, a collection of joints, levers, and hinges that passively do what the muscles tell them to do. They do not need to be in mint condition to perform their simple, passive functions. As an example, I have a cracked meniscus in my knee. I would never have known it had I not had an MRI for a different reason. When the radiologist saw the meniscal tear, he asked me if I had been having any pain. I told him I had not, nor had I any limitation in my functional capacity or range of motion. He found that hard to believe. His parting comment to me was that if I had been having pain, surgery would have been recommended. Fortunately, the muscles that track the course of the sciatic nerve down to my knee were healthy enough not to have been causing nerve irritation, or I might have had knee surgery for nothing! So if you or someone you know is suffering from acute or chronic musculoskeletal pain, beware of the temptation to think that surgery or some other invasive procedure for a structural abnormality in the area of the pain will solve the problem.

Thankfully, there is a way to fully restore the health of sickened, spastic muscles. That's good news for all of us because every one of us, from the weekend couch potato to the health-conscious fitness buff have some spastic muscle. Though we may be unaware of its presence, it is surely there, slowly growing and placing us at ever-increasing risk for pain, injury, and disease as we age.

Other treatment options for chronic musculoskeletal pain

Before we get into the details of the definitive treatment for chronic musculoskeletal pain, let's talk about some of the other treatments that are available. One of the first and most commonly recommended treatments is medication. While there are times when medication is the only effective means of achieving immediate pain relief, the duration of its use should be limited, and it should not be used as a substitute for treating the underlying problem. Yet because the cause of acute and chronic musculoskeletal pain is still misunderstood by most physicians, far too many patients continue to be treated with far too many medications for far too long. Ironically, many patients who come to depend on pain medication are later reprimanded or even dropped by the doctors who prescribed the medication in the first place. In essence, patients are blamed when medication fails to correct a problem that it cannot possibly correct. Muscle relaxants, anti-inflammatories, and narcotics might provide temporary pain relief, but rather than correcting the underlying abnormality, they can mask it and even cause it to worsen over time. Many of these medications can also be habit-forming, thus complicating the clinical picture by creating drug dependence.

Alongside medication, the most widely recommended treatment for musculoskeletal pain is physical therapy. On the positive side, physical therapy does target the problem tissue--muscle, and if begun soon after the onset of symptoms, proper stretching and strengthening can potentially flush enough lactic acid out of the superficial layers of tight muscles to relieve symptoms despite the fact that the core of hypertonicity remains. But even if the therapist and the patient understand the physiology of the problem, it can be difficult to gauge what intensity, duration, and frequency of exercise will help rid the muscles of lactic acid without overwhelming them and locking more lactic acid in. As discussed earlier, spastic muscle, whether it is causing back pain, neck pain, knee pain, hip pain, or some other pain, is caught in a vicious cycle of spasm, and that spasm can be worsened by an exercise regimen or even one movement that overwhelms the affected muscle or muscles.

The means by which physical therapy is more likely to be effective in reducing pain and improving function is through its effect on the muscle tissue that is still healthy. Proper loosening and strengthening can potentially condition enough healthy muscle to compensate for the muscle that is hypertonic. As strength and flexibility improve, functionality improves, and some of the stress may be taken off the hypertonic tissue, which in turn can reduce the symptoms of nerve irritation that it is causing. Selecting the right exercises and finding the right balance of intensity, duration, and frequency is crucial so as not to push compensatory muscles into spasm or push the muscles that are causing the symptoms deeper into spasm. In most advanced cases, such a perfect balance is virtually impossible to achieve on a continuous basis.

Another common treatment for musculoskeletal pain is steroid injections. The goal of treatment is to reduce the inflammation around the structural abnormality that is presumed to be causing the symptoms. In the case of disc-related sciatica, for instance, the injection is aimed at reducing local inflammation so as to reduce irritation of spinal nerve roots that are believed to be impinged by the protruding disc. But if there really were inflammation, and that inflammation were causing the symptoms, wouldn't whatever was causing the inflammation cause the symptoms to return after the injection had worn off? Logically yes; but that's not what we see. Instead, we see a cumulative lasting effect of steroid injections in those patients who respond to the treatment. In fact the standard procedure is to give a short series of injections with decreasing frequency--three or four in all. So how do we explain what we observe clinically? The answer is that for some individuals, the procedure itself and the irritant effect of the steroid stimulates enough of an endorphin response to have a powerful pain-relieving effect. The endorphin response is even greater for more invasive procedures like laminectomies, cartilage repairs, and joint replacements, thus explaining the apparent success of these procedures. However, none of these operations do anything to restore the health of hypertonic muscle. The notion that an invasive procedure in itself can relieve symptoms was put to the test in a recent study involving knee surgery.[4] Patients were randomly divided into two groups, one receiving real surgery and the other receiving sham surgery, in which an equally invasive procedure was performed without an actual tissue repair. Interestingly, there was no statistical difference in the success rate between the two groups. Although we cannot rule out the placebo effect, we need look no further than the endorphin effect to explain the results.

Endorphins are the body's natural pain-killers. Their existence was discovered after World War II, when research was done to investigate how severely wounded soldiers, though conscious and not in shock, could feel no pain and even undergo surgical repair of their injuries without anesthesia. What researchers discovered was that the body produces a group of chemicals that bind to pain receptors in the brain even more perfectly than the synthetic pain-killer morphine. These were naturally occurring (internal) morphines; hence the term "endorphins." Because they are made by the body, endorphins are hundreds of times more powerful than morphine at masking pain, they are continuously available, and they produce no side effects. What this means is that the body can be in a great deal of distress without the individual knowing it. In fact, the individual can feel really good because endorphins can also create a sense of euphoria. It is for this "high" that drug addicts abuse morphine and its better-known derivative--heroin. Over time, their use of the drug causes the body to stop producing endorphins. The excruciating pain of withdrawal that an addict experiences when he or she suddenly stops using heroin gives you an idea of how powerful endorphins are.

The combination of the endorphin response to steroid injections and the thought that something is being done to remedy the problem can, for many patients, provide satisfactory relief. Pain relief can, in turn, facilitate a return to normal activities that can partially recondition muscle and prevent the further development of hypertonic spasm. Notwithstanding, steroid injections should preferably be avoided because of the risk of infection and the damaging effect that they have on the tissues into which they are injected. Of greatest concern are spinal injections, which can cause a central nervous system infection or nerve damage as the needle is passed into the epidural space. The risk of these complications is small, but even when a series of epidural injections does provide pain relief without any complications, it does not correct the underlying problem of hypertonic spasm.

The same is true for shoulder, hip, and knee pain thought due to osteoarthritis. Here again, steroid injections are often used to relieve pain that is presumed to be caused by inflammation--in this case created by bone-on-bone irritation within the joint. In many cases, one or a series of injections does alleviate the pain, but the effect often lasts much longer than would be predicted from a purely anti-inflammatory effect. The other inconsistency is that patients are often told to remain active, a recommendation that directly contradicts the theory that the pain is caused by bone-on-bone irritation. Nevertheless, those patients who do remain active generally fair better than those who do not. In fact, some of those who remain active will not need further treatment. And why is that? Because once again, the pain is usually not caused by a structural abnormality but by hypertonic muscle, and movement benefits the healthy portion of the muscles that are hypertonic.

Another treatment, commonly recommended for neck and lower back pain, is spinal traction. The idea behind traction is to passively stretch the spine in an effort to draw a bulging disc back into the intervertebral space so as to take pressure off an impinged nerve root. Some therapists and treatment centers even claim that traction can facilitate the healing of a herniated disc in such a way that the disc permanently stops irritating nerve roots. Here again, the treatment is targeted at the structural abnormality rather than the true source of the symptoms. To be sure, the pain and, in some cases, numbness and tingling down an arm or leg is in fact due to nerve impingement, but the culprit is generally not the disc but spastic muscle.

Intervertebral discs are donut-shaped fibrous structures that are firmly attached between the vertically stacked vertebrae of the spinal column. They are composed of a tough fibrocartilaginous outer portion called the *annulus fibrosus* and a soft central portion called the *nucleus pulposus* that consists mostly of water, collagen, and polysaccharide gel. Discs allow the vertebrae to swivel without rubbing against each other and act as shock-absorbers for the boney spine. The prevailing theory is that cracks and tears in the outer ring allow soft material from the central portion of the disc to squeeze out like toothpaste. The common belief is that this material then irritates local nerve roots, thus leading to pain and other symptoms that are associated with a herniated disc.

While it is true that intervertebral discs do start out having a well hydrated center, discs lose blood supply as we age, causing the soft central portion to dry out and harden. By the age of thirty, there is already mild to moderate disc degeneration (drying out), and by middle age, which is when the majority of disc herniations are diagnosed, the disc is as hard as rubber, having the look and feel of a small hockey puck. So even if a disc were to crack or tear, there isn't much to squeeze out. That's why jet fighter pilots can pull out of steep dives that place hundreds of pounds of pressure on their spines without doing any damage to their discs.[5]

As discussed earlier, more detailed studies conducted within the last five years have found little correlation between MRI pathology and either the patient's symptoms or course of improvement.[2,3] Of no less importance is the devastating effect that the disc theory has on patients psychologically and behaviorally. When patients are told that they have a disc problem, they come away fearing that if they merely twist, bend, or lift something, they could make their problem worse. So they naturally begin to restrict their activities. But from what we have discussed about muscle health and the ubiquitous phenomenon of hypertonic spasm, we know that restricting one's activities could potentially create a vicious cycle of declining function from which there could be no escape.

Much more relevant than intermittent loading of the spine is the effect of the continuous loading that chronically contracted muscle has on the flexible discs and near-by nerves. Contracted and stiff as they are, spastic muscles place continuous pressure on the discs, causing them to bulge or even tear. The tight muscles also trap, squeeze, and rub against local nerves to the point of creating symptoms. To get a sense of this, try grasping two of your fingers from the opposite hand and squeeze gently. Notice that you do not feel any discomfort. That's because your hand, like a healthy resting muscle, is relatively relaxed. Now begin to squeeze your fingers harder and harder. Notice that after a few moments, both your fingers and the hand squeezing them begin to feel uncomfortable. Now imagine continuing to squeeze really hard without ever stopping! You can bet that sooner or later, the nerves in your hand, your wrist, and your fingers will really start to complain. That is what happens when you tweak a muscle into acute spasm. Over time, the accumulation of trapped lactic acid causes the muscle to become tighter and tighter, which in turn irritates local nerves. That's why the injury, which is really nothing more than a muscle having been pushed beyond its reserve capacity, often does not start causing symptoms until the morning after. If allowed to remain in an overly contracted state, an acute spasm can turn into hypertonic spasm and become permanent. When that happens, it's like continuing to squeeze your fingers harder and harder for the rest of your life! In such cases, the only thing that prevents the pain from becoming overwhelming is the production of endorphins.

To illustrate this point, I have a herniated disc in my lower back that was believed to be causing sciatic nerve symptoms down my right leg. As the months passed, the pain was gradually subsiding, but I could feel the muscles becoming tighter and tighter. I was told that thirty to forty thrice weekly sessions of spinal traction (mechanical stretching) would rehydrate and heal the disc, take the pressure off my sciatic nerve, and completely alleviate my symptoms. Sounds great, right? Well even after fifty sessions of spinal traction, I was no better. Some of the other patients were reporting improvement, but unlike me, those who were improving had been experiencing pain in the muscles that were being stretched; namely, their necks and backs. So if all of us had been having nerve pain from a herniated disc, then why wasn't I getting better? No one had an answer. I can only conclude that the mechanism of pain relief for those who had been improving was not decompression of the nerve root but the antispasmodic effect of stretching their tight muscles--a benefit that I was not receiving because my spastic muscles were not in my back but in my leg, and my leg was not being stretched. In any case, I stopped going, but I did not stop investigating. By God's grace, I eventually discovered the phenomenon of hypertonic spasm and its treatment. That's when I finally started to get better.

Another common treatment for musculoskeletal pain is chiropractic. As with PT, there are numerous forms and techniques, but the theory behind all of them is that misalignments in the vertebral column called *subluxations* can cause nerves to be pinched at the point where they exit the spine, thereby creating nerve pain and dysfunction. The purpose of the "adjustment" is to relieve the pain and optimize nerve function by restoring spinal alignment. However, the theory behind chiropractic is errant in two respects. First, there is a misunderstanding about how spinal misalignments occur. Chiropractors are taught that poor posture and physical trauma such as bumps, falls, and various injuries can force vertebrae out of alignment, as if the spine were a stack of casino chips that can easily be disrupted. In reality, the spine is quite flexible and when distorted is immediately pulled back into neutral position by the muscles that keep it in alignment. Thus, if a subluxation were present, it would not be due to a bump or fall but to an imbalance in muscle tone. The other error in chiropractic theory is that spinal misalignments adversely affect nerve function. In an elegant test of chiropractic's subluxation theory, Dr. Edmund Crelin, a professor of anatomy at the Yale University School of Medicine, analyzed and dissected human spines to see if distortions in spinal alignment would crowd any of the spinal nerves as they exit the spine. He concluded that "for impingements to occur, ligaments would have to be ripped apart and bones broken."[6,7] Thus, he demonstrated that the theory behind chiropractic is erroneous. Notwithstanding, chiropractic adjustments do seem to help some patients feel better. The short-term improvement is most likely due to a temporary increase in flexibility and endorphin production in response to the stimulating effect of the adjustment. But because chiropractic adjustments do not restore normal function to hypertonic muscle, maintenance therapy is necessary. Those who remain interested in seeking chiropractic care should choose a chiropractor who uses an Activator, ProAdjuster, or other such device because there is a risk of serious injury when the hands are used to forcibly "crack" the spine.

There are a number of other modalities that claim to be effective in the treatment of musculoskeletal pain, such as acupuncture, craniosacral therapy, muscle stimulators, and various forms of massage. Though these and related techniques do help some patients, they do not yield consistent results and can, in some cases, make symptoms worse. As an example, I was treated with a direct current stimulator called ARP (Accelerated Recovery Performance), which significantly improved my overly contracted hamstring. However, a subsequent treatment by the same provider using the same instrument made the spasm worse. Sometime later, I tried deep tissue massage with a another therapist. The first two sessions seemed to have helped somewhat, but the third nearly crippled me for two weeks! I experienced inconsistent results with a number of other treatment modalities as well. All that changed when I came across the work of Dr. Thomas Griner and KANON myotherapy.

+ + +

CHAPTER 6

APPLICATION OF THE TECHNIQUE

Because hypertonic muscle is hardened muscle, only the superficial layer of the spastic core can be reached by KANON stimulation. The deeper layers are protected from stimulation until the outermost layer of spasticity is relieved. Hence, hypertonic muscle can only be released one layer at a time. The process is like peeling an onion, or more accurately, like an archeological dig because these are not so much layers of individual muscle fibers as they are layers of trauma. As such, the release of one layer might free up more or less muscle tissue than another. As each layer of spasm is released, more of the muscle regains flexibility and function. The more penetrating the therapy, the more apt the muscle is to remain healthy because it has regained that much more blood flow, functional capacity, and healthy reserve. With persistent application of the technique, the bulk of the muscle can potentially be restored to health, thereby enabling a person to feel like and do the things they did when they were younger.

In actual practice, the KANON technique is rarely applied to only one muscle. Even if the pain or other symptoms seem to be localized to one particular area or one muscle, we must remember that muscles work in synergistic groups and, thus, are likely to have become hypertonic in groups. So whatever has happened to one muscle is likely to have happened to others in the group. Hence, the therapy usually needs to target all the muscles in a symptomatic area and sometimes even distant muscles.

KANON myotherapy is truly a partnership between the patient and the therapist because the choice of where to focus the treatment as well as the intensity and duration of the treatment requires continuous input from the patient. After taking a history, the therapist will carefully search for areas of tight, spastic muscle. However, some muscles that seem less involved to the therapist might feel more involved to the patient. That's an important guide to the therapist. The therapist also needs feedback about the pressure being applied by the BioPulser® and the length of stimulation of a given area. Finally, patient feedback about the recovery time of each treatment is important in guiding the length of time to the next treatment.

To obtain maximum benefit from a treatment, the patient should relax as much as possible, particularly in the area where the therapist is working. Voluntary muscle tension tends to prevent both the fingertip massage and the BioPulser® from stimulating the nerve beds that relay corrective feedback to the cerebellum. As a general rule, problem areas will be the focus of treatment, and with the 2013 upgrade of the BioPulser®, any point on the muscle can be pulsed continuously for several minutes or more without overwhelming the tissue. Even so, feedback from both the patient and the muscle is important in helping the therapist correctly apply the treatment and avoid over-stimulating the tissue. As one who has been successfully treated with the KANON technique, I found that the more relaxing the treatment, the more effective it was. Treatment is most pleasurable when the unwanted stretch reflex, which causes muscles to tighten rather than relax, is avoided. Through years of research, Dr. Griner found that muscles can tolerate a static pressure of no more than about six ounces before they fire the stretch reflex. The firing threshold increases to a pound or a pound-and-a-half if the muscle is massaged across the grain, which is why the KANON practitioner always massages the muscle that way.

In most cases, areas of hypertonic muscle are so hard that they are difficult to massage effectively without triggering the stretch reflex or creating excessive inflammation. That's where the BioPulser® becomes a complementary necessity to the fingertip massage. The BioPulser® is scientifically engineered to deliver a strong biocompatible nerve response that is highly effective in relaxing hypertonic muscle. The tapping of the machine creates a pulsatile wave that causes the muscle to relax. Note that the BioPulser® does not break up hardened muscle the way a jack hammer breaks up concrete or the way deep tissue massage attempts to loosen muscle. To attempt such a thing would accomplish just the opposite because the heavy pressure would trigger the stretch reflex, which causes the muscle to contract. Muscle hardness is a neurologically-driven fixed state of over-contraction that must be precisely stimulated in order to relax. If the BioPulser® is used too forcefully, the muscle could become even more spastic. The BioPulser® is different from other vibrating devices in that the tapping speed and frequency are precisely calibrated to avoid overloading nerve circuits and triggering the stretch reflex. The intensity of the vibration can be adjusted both by changing the thickness of the washers on the neck of the pulsating head and by varying the angle at which the instrument is held against the body. An added advantage of the BioPulser® is that it is easier to master than the fingertip massage technique and causes less inflammation. It can also access muscles that are inaccessible to massage, and its therapeutic effect is more diffuse and more penetrating. However, there are benefits from the skilled application of the fingertip technique that the BioPulser® does not necessarily provide. Therefore, the BioPulser is best used in combination with fingertip massage rather than as a substitute for it. In most cases, and especially in severe cases where there is little or no healthy tissue, the BioPulser® can be used alone until enough progress is made to add fingertip massage.

Since the goal of therapy is to flush toxins out of hypertonic muscle, drinking plenty of water before and after a treatment is very important. As a general rule, drinking smaller quantities at regular intervals is more effective at maintaining good hydration than drinking larger quantities more sporadically because the body quickly excretes the excess fluid. A good indicator of whether you are staying well-hydrated is the color of your urine. Ideally, it should remain light yellow or colorless. A helpful detoxification hint is to include fresh vegetable juices and whole fresh fruit in your diet.

The treatment itself, whether it be the hand massage or the BioPulser®, creates inflammation, which temporarily makes susceptible muscle tissue more prone to spasm and reverting to the hypertonic state. Therefore, strenuous exercise should be avoided for several days after a treatment. If the lower body muscles feel tight immediately after being worked on, it is advisable to lie down for awhile to allow them to loosen before bearing weight. While at rest, staying well-hydrated and moving the legs periodically will facilitate detoxification by stimulating circulation without driving up lactic acid production. In general, one can expect three phases of recovery from a treatment: an initial loosening of the muscles during the first hour post-treatment; followed by several days of increased susceptibility to spasm due to inflammation; and finally a further loosening of the muscles with increased range of motion and functional capacity. The total recovery time from a treatment is typically correlated with the effectiveness of the treatment; the longer it takes to fully recover from a treatment, the more effective the treatment. The average recovery time is about seven to ten days, though complete tissue repair actually takes about three to four weeks.

As muscles begin to soften in response to treatment, pain and other symptoms of nerve irritation will begin to resolve; however, the perception of this will be affected by several factors. First, endorphins, the body's natural pain killers, are likely to be very active leading up to the start of treatment. As such, they are likely to have been masking some of the pain that the treatment is intended to resolve. As treatment progresses, changes in the body's endorphin response might unmask some of the pain that had been there all along. In addition, areas of spastic muscle might become more tender as the muscles begin to soften in response to treatment. Also, new areas of pain might crop up as the body learns to redistribute forces in a healthier, more balanced proportion. As my own treatment allowed me to start walking longer distances, my knees and feet began to hurt because they had grown unaccustomed to such stresses during the years that I was unable to function. In addition, creaking sounds that seemed to have been emanating from joints but which were actually created by the movement of tight muscles and tendons gradually disappeared. Also, my skin regained sensitivity that had been altered by the constant irritation of associated nerves and the production of endorphins. In some individuals, a skin rash might appear temporarily as histamine is released from spastic muscle tissue. There might be other changes as well, but in general, change is good; it's the evidence that progress is being made.

The goal of a series of treatments is to release one spastic layer of muscle at a time, a process that allows the therapy to penetrate deeper and deeper into the muscle and thus restore more and more of its healthy function. To accomplish this, treatment sessions need to be spaced far enough apart to allow the muscle to respond to the treatment but not so far that the newly released tissue lapses back into spasm. Typically, that means sessions spaced a week or two apart. As more and more tissue is released, circulation improves, making the newly released tissue increasingly resistant to lapsing back into chronic spasm. With continued treatment, the normal function and reserve capacity of the muscles is restored, and treatment sessions can be spaced farther apart. The length of a course of treatment will depend on the individual's goals and lifestyle. The longer and more penetrating the therapy, the wider the range of activities the individual will be able to preform and the more resistant the muscles will be to becoming hypertonic again. Once the treatment goal is met, treatment can either be stopped or reduced to occasional maintenance sessions. I recommend occasional maintenance not because the therapeutic effect is lost over time but because, in the absence of significant lifestyle changes, the same factors that caused the muscles to become hypertonic in the past are apt to cause them to become hypertonic again. We will discuss changes in exercise routine and daily habits that can prevent relapse and progression of hypertonic spasm.

Beware that releasing hypertonic muscle is only half the battle. The other half is to strengthen the newly released tissue. Depending on the duration and extent of the hypertonicity, the newly released muscle might be weak because during the time that it was hypertonic, it had neither been functioning properly nor receiving healthy blood flow. Recall that hypertonic muscles choke off their own blood supply, which leaves them chronically congested with toxins while at the same time being chronically overworked because they are chronically over-contracted. What's more, the reduced physical activity that is often associated with chronic pain tends to decondition the healthy portion of hypertonic muscles as well as synergist (helper) muscles. Depending on how deconditioned these muscles are, the simple act of picking up something weighty or even prolonged standing or walking could drive the newly released tissue back into spasm. Hence, a vital part of therapy is to recondition both the treated muscles and the associated weakened muscles. This must be done gradually and in the right way to prevent the exercise itself from causing a recurrence of hypertonic spasm.

The type and intensity of exercise one can do between treatments will depend on the extent and severity of the hypertonus. It will also depend on the level of fitness of the individual prior to the onset of symptoms, the length of time physical activity had been restricted prior to the start of treatment, how much healthy tissue the hypertonic muscles have, which muscles are affected, the relative distribution of forces during exercise, and the predominant muscle fiber type of the individual. Those with a predominance of fast-twitch fibers are both more prone to developing hypertonic spasm and slower to respond to treatment because fast-twitch muscle is the predominant lactic acid producer. Fast-twitch muscle also mediates the stretch reflex, which works contrary to the goal of treatment because it causes muscles to forcefully contract, thereby driving up lactic acid production. Most persons have a fairly even balance of slow and fast-twitch muscle. If you are in the minority of individuals who have predominantly slow-twitch fibers, you will tend to walk, run, and move slower but with greater endurance than those with predominantly fast-twitch fibers. You are also likely to have less muscle bulk and less ability to generate explosive force than your fast-twitch counterparts. Long-distance runners tend to have a predominance of slow-twitch muscle, whereas most other competitive athletes tend to have a predominance of fast-twitch muscle.

With so many variables involved, there is going to be some uncertainty as to how much and which type of exercises are best for an individual. As a general rule, we want to select exercises that maximize circulation and minimize lactic acid production. As a swimmer and avid golfer, I found that once I had progressed far enough in recovery, combining swimming with golf was a great way to do just that. As a routine, I would go for a brief swim to loosen up my muscles in preparation for the back bends and hip movements in golf that would further increase my range of motion and loosen up my muscles even more. I was also mindful that overdoing it could cause the buildup of too much lactic acid, and so I chose to ride in a golf cart rather than walk the whole course. Also, I would return to the pool for a brief swim after the round to facilitate the removal of the lactic acid I had accumulated playing golf. Whatever your exercise interests might be, the golden rule is to take it slow, and listen to your body. As each successive layer of hypertonic muscle is released through repeated treatments, range of motion, strength, and endurance will naturally increase. Your responsibility is to take what your body gives you and work with it in moderation. As your recovery progresses, avoid the temptation to jump back into strenuous activities because some muscles or groups of muscles might still be too spastic to keep up with muscles that have regained greater flexibly and strength. If overtaxed, the tighter muscles could be driven back into spasm. Patience, moderation, and discernment in this regard will minimize the risk of setbacks during the delicate transition back to health. Also remember that slow movements with low resistance will help prevent the overproduction of lactic acid. In severe cases of lower extremity hypertonus, water exercises and short-distance walking can be a bridge to longer distance walking and more strenuous activities. This will help ensure that you strengthen the muscles without overwhelming them and causing them to lock back up. We'll talk more about healthy exercise in the next chapter.

Although KANON non-invasive has an extraordinarily high success rate, the rate of recovery is difficult to predict because of the many variables involved. In addition to the those previously mentioned, the severity and duration of the condition, the experience of the therapist, and the constitution of the patient are important in determining the rate of recovery. Some patients' muscles are ready to bust out and revitalize with just a little help, while others are more resistant to change. Although long-standing conditions tend to require a proportionately greater number of treatments, there are times when a chronic condition will respond more swiftly than one of recent onset. The treatment response can vary even for a given individual, as some layers of spasm are larger than others and when released will give way to a larger jump in improvement. Even if a layer of spasm is not fully released during a treatment session, progress in that direction has likely been made, as some of the lactic acid is likely to have been flushed out of the congested muscles. Regardless of the severity or duration of the condition, the decisive factor in determining the outcome of treatment is the persistence and commitment of the patient and the therapist to keep working on it until the desired degree of improvement has been achieved.

Although KANON myotherapy can, in theory, completely restore the health of hypertonic muscle, to do so is generally unnecessary because we need only release enough spastic muscle to alleviate pain and restore normal function. Those who wish to return to more demanding activities or restore more reserve capacity will need a longer course of treatment.

Currently, the biggest treatment challenge is the lack of KANON practitioners in most states across the country. Word about this revolutionary treatment is still in its fledgling stages, and it may be some time before the treatment is available in your area. If you live in the Chicago area, you can contact Sharon Drewett at sharondrewett78@gmail.com or by phone at (312) 371-7255. Ms. Drewett has several years of experience with both the BioPulser® and the fingertip massage techniques. If you live elsewhere in the United States, you can contact Dr. Thomas Griner at kanonbio@gmail.com.

Even if it is not possible to see a KANON practitioner, the BioPulser® Signature Series is available for purchase at www.biopulser.com. With the help of the principles discussed in this book, you could use the instrument on yourself, although it would be easier and more effective if a therapist or trainer were to use it on you. There would be a learning curve for anyone who is inexperienced, but patience and persistence should lead to the desired benefit. The treatment can even be done with a spouse, family member, or friend if they are willing to dedicate themselves to helping you. Those interested should read Dr. Griner's book entitled What's Really Wrong With You?[8] and visit his website www.kanonbio.com.

+ + +

CHAPTER 7

PRINCIPLES OF HEALTHY EXERCISE

We have reached a new era in the world of fitness. Unlike in the past when young people and athletes were the only ones in the gym, today people of all ages and walks of life are looking to get fit. From housewives to business executives and school teachers to aging seniors, it seems that everyone is jumping on the fitness bandwagon. To fan the flame, we are bombarded with adds, articles, and CDs on fitness, not to mention the limitless types of equipment that are advertised to meet our fitness needs.

But did you know that exercise can be as bad for your health as being an overweight couch potato? To be sure, exercise has an enormous potential to optimize health; but in order to reap that benefits without doing harm, we need to understand the principles by which exercise enhances mental and physical health. A human being is mind, body, and spirit. Therefore, let us begin with a discussion of the mind as it pertains to healthy exercise and follow with a discussion of muscle function as it pertains to the general health of the body and the development of a healthy exercise routine.

On a mental and emotional level, exercise can be relaxing and rejuvenating; but to fully experience those benefits, it must be undertaken with the right attitude and under the right conditions. To understand how exercise affects the mind, let us first review the anatomy of the mind. I had been practicing medicine for over ten years before I was able to piece together the anatomy of this most complex and fascinating part of our being. Through a combination of

43

psychiatry, neurology, spirituality, and the experiences of my patients as well as my own, I came to the realization that the mind is not one thing or another but a dialogue; it is a dialogue between the brain and the psyche or "soul."

You see, your brain is not you. Rather, it is an organ that you use together with the rest of your body to interact with the physical world. Notice that you do not say, I am brain; or, I am body. Instead you say, this is my brain, and this is my body. So if your brain and your body are not you, then who are you? The answer is that YOU are a living being, a soul complete with emotion, intellect, and will. The brain has none of these attributes; it is merely a computer in your head that works for you like a laptop computer. It's a "head-top" if you will. And just like your personal computer, your brain processes and stores everything that you--the soul--tell it to.

So now that we understand what the brain is, and we understand what the soul is, we can understand the mind as the dialogue between the two. As the soul attempts to think, he or she creates subtle energy fields that influence the brain, and the brain creates complementary fields that influence the soul. This brain activity is part of what neurologists read on an electrical recording made by attaching tiny electrodes to the scalp. It is also one of the methods used to determine whether a patient who is in a coma is alive or dead because the brain can no longer process information, or "think" once the soul leaves the body. That having been said, we are ready to discuss how exercise affects the mind.

When undertaken with the right attitude under the right conditions, exercise allows the soul to take a break from intellectualizing and focus on simple movements of the body. The mental simplicity of this reduces the dialogue between the soul and the brain, thus giving both of them a rest. This "meditative" aspect of exercise is one of the ways that it rejuvenates the mind because the quieter our brain is, the more relaxed and rested we feel. That's one of the reasons we should set our worldly cares aside when we are working out.

The other way in which exercise rejuvenates the mind is by boosting the production of serotonin, dopamine, and norepinephrine. These neurotransmitters are the body's natural antidepressants. Exercise also boosts the production of endorphins, which, as discussed previously, are the body's natural pain killers. Together these "feel-good" chemicals create a mild euphoria that summates with the meditative aspect of exercise to make life's challenges seem a lot more manageable after a physically vigorous but emotionally relaxing workout.

Deriving these mental and emotional benefits from exercise probably sounds like a simple matter, and it would be were it not for life's constant demands, misconceptions, and negative influences. A wide range of circumstances, beliefs, and attitudes can jeopardize the mental and emotional benefits of exercise by causing us to hurry through a workout, overdo a workout, exercise too frequently, or never exercise at all.

Hurrying through a workout detracts from the meditative aspect of exercise because it is usually accompanied by stressful thoughts and concerns that get the brain worked up. It also increases the risk of injury because the mind is preoccupied with things other than form, deep breathing, and other important aspects of a healthy exercise technique. Also, from a neurochemical standpoint, emotional stress causes chemical changes that counter the beneficial effects of exercise. It also prevents muscle growth by stimulating the release of corticotropins, which decrease amino acid uptake and protein synthesis by muscle tissue.

Prolonging a workout can have the same negative effect on the mind as hurrying through a workout. As previously stated, exercise boosts the production of the feel-good neurotransmitters serotonin, dopamine, and norepinephrine. However, over-training can drive up the production of a derivative of norepinephrine called epinephrine. Epinephrine, more commonly known as *adrenaline*, is a "fight or flight" hormone that can create irritability and even panic attacks. Thus, the inordinate drive to achieve fast results or attempt to pack a whole week's workout into a single visit to the gym can end up backfiring emotionally as well as physically. The same phenomenon can occur if exercise becomes too frequent because a fatigued body is an irritable one. A fatigued body is also more susceptible to colds and flus because the immune system is drained of energy, though one might not feel drained when the endorphin level is high. The impatient and the overzealous would do well to remember that the strain of exercise breaks down the body; the physical gains are made during the recovery phase. Hence the importance of moderation, ample rest, and a steady stream of nutrients during the recovery phase between workouts.

A big challenge on the mental side of exercise is sticking to a routine. Whether it be a pressing project at work, a time-consuming relationship, or just plain laziness, life has a way of encroaching on our exercise routine. Personally I found that with the cessation of exercise, the antidepressant effect can be lost in as little as two to three weeks. Some might say even sooner than that. From a medical-psychiatric standpoint, I would say that it depends on the neurochemical constitution of one's brain. For some individuals, boosting serotonin, norepinephrine, and dopamine, like prescription antidepressants, has a more immediate effect than for others. Be that as it may, the antidepressant effect is rapidly lost with breaks in one's exercise routine, particularly the more "aerobic" component of the routine. Part of the problem is that when this occurs, one usually fails to realize what's happening. One commonly begins to dwell on some small problem or negative thought until it becomes a big one. That's because the exercise hormones stimulate positive pathways in the brain until their levels drop. As they drop, we begin to see the glass of life more as half empty than half full. But because both ways of seeing it are technically correct, we can fail to recognize that our perspective is changing. What's more, even if we were to recognize that our perspective had changed, we might not realize that it was caused by a discontinuation of our exercise routine and the associated loss of antidepressant effect.

Many years ago, I had temporarily discontinued the aerobic part of my exercise routine because running was starting to cause lower back pain. Though I had continued regular strength-training, I started to feel like there was a black cloud over my head. As hard as I tried to explain the feeling of worry, I could not find any logical explanation; the circumstances of my life were no different than they had been when I stopped running three weeks earlier. Because my back was starting to feel better, I resumed jogging on alternate days. The first day back to running did nothing to improve my mental outlook. But about fifteen minutes into the next scheduled run, I felt the warmth of the sun break through the dark emotional cloud! By the end of my thirty-minute run,

I found myself feeling good again. However, had a real life crisis occurred during the break in my exercise routine, I naturally would have assumed it to be the sole cause of my excessive worry.

What makes it even more confusing is that emotional stress can partially mask the mood-lifting effects of exercise, causing the world to look dark even when regular exercise is doing its job neurochemically. This can cause us to underestimate the emotional benefit of exercise and allow stressful circumstances to pull us off our exercise routine. Later, when the crises has ended, we would then be more likely to go on feeling as though the clouds remain simply because we never returned to exercise. This not only leaves a persistent shadow on our emotional outlook but it also leaves us emotionally vulnerable to the next potential crisis both because we have stopped exercising and because we have lost the neurochemical momentum that regular exercise creates. This in turn makes us a set-up for developing a mood disorder because prolonged emotional stress and negative thinking can cause long-lasting changes in brain chemistry that may ultimately require medical treatment. Then again, some individuals have chronic emotional disorders and other abnormalities of brain chemistry that may require ongoing treatment even under the best of circumstances. However, that does not detract from the importance of regular exercise; if anything, it adds to it.

Exercise also produces both an immediate and long-term increase in stamina and productivity. Ordinarily, one hour of moderate exercise can provide up to three extra hours of productive wake time per twenty-four hour period. Although that benefit is rapidly lost upon discontinuation of regular exercise, the long-term effect is not. Thus, discontinuation of regular exercise will result in an immediate step down in stamina and productivity, but the second step down can be delayed for long periods, sometimes even years, depending upon how much reserve capacity has been acquired by adhering to an effective exercise routine. So the idea that one's busy schedule does not allow time for exercise is a paradox. In reality, just the opposite is true: making time for exercise will buy even more time to meet the demands of a busy schedule. Moderate regular exercise also strengthens the immune system and reduces the recovery time from injury or disease, both of which reduce the risk of failing to meet one's obligations.

This leads to a word of caution. The transition back to exercise after a lengthy break in routine can be a dangerous one. The mind tends to remember what the body can do far better than the body does. As an example, I had maintained a comprehensive exercise routine for several years before I got busy writing my first book. One of the factors that allowed me to slip out of my routine was the abundance of stamina I had stored up from years of steady exercise and a healthy diet. Anyhow, as I was getting back to exercise after a seven-year break, I injured myself doing a familiar exercise. My mind was ready, but my body was not. This applies to aerobic exercise as well as strength-training. Any break in routine for more than a few weeks is deserving of special caution. Upon returning to exercise, one should err on the side of doing too little rather than too much until the body clearly demonstrates that it is ready for more.

Then again, most people face an even greater challenge than sticking to an exercise routine. For millions of Americans, the biggest problem is one of just getting started. In most cases, the hurdle is primarily mental, as the mind becomes overwhelmed with thoughts about the burden of regular exercise for the rest of one's life. Most beginners imagine themselves starting off doing what others do as part of their advanced routine and, among other things, can't even see how it can fit into their busy schedule. Clearly, that kind of thinking can leave one feeling too overwhelmed to start anything!

The good news is that regular exercise is not nearly as difficult as most people imagine. It's really just a matter of getting into the habit. That's why the secret to getting started is to begin gradually; and when I say gradually, I mean just a few minutes of walking or strengthening per day. Clearly that should fit into anyone's schedule! One can also make some health-conscious changes at work, such as using the stairwell rather than the elevator and standing up to stretch periodically rather than remaining seated for long periods of time. Changes like these might seem insignificant from a physical standpoint, but they are not; and from a mental standpoint, they are huge. The trick is to become exercise-conscious without getting scared off by taking on too much too fast. Once the idea of exercise becomes firmly rooted in one's mind and some of the early benefits are realized, the habit will continue to grow. Of course, those with known medical conditions and the elderly should discuss any planned exercises with their doctors. Some forms of exercise might be more advisable than others, and some limits of intensity might need to be observed.

Once it is established as a routine, regular exercise becomes, among other things, a tangible accomplishment that helps keep one motivated regardless of what the day may bring. This benefit makes early morning exercise ideal. Early morning is also the time when the body is normally at peak energy due to a cyclic rise in growth hormone and cortisol. The early morning spike in energy is an adaptive advantage because, having been stagnant all night, the body has accumulated a toxic load by morning and is in need of exercise to flush the toxins out of the system, including those that have accumulated in muscle tissue.

Besides making us feel better, regular exercise helps us look better, and that alone can be a powerful motivator to establish a healthy exercise routine. Added to this is the knowledge that what we eat can either contribute to or undo what we are trying to accomplish through exercise. The idea that a soft drink or candy bar could undo all the calorie-burning we just did with a healthy workout is usually enough to persuade one to take a pass and prepare a healthy snack.

The secret to establishing a healthy diet is to understand that we learn to like whatever we eat on a regular basis. Hence, we need not struggle to make healthy foods more palatable, nor do we need to deprive ourselves of what we like to eat. We just need to start following a diet that is ideally suited to our health and fitness needs, and then continue doing it until we learn to like it. I personally started doing this several years ago and found it to be the best kept secret to the whole diet problem. All my life I had enjoyed eating cereal and an occasional egg or pancake breakfast. Then one day while my uncle was visiting, I saw him eating a plate of mixed vegetables, olives, and cheese for breakfast. To me it looked tasteless in comparison to what I was used to eating; worse yet, I detested olives. Yet I could not argue with the fact that it was a healthful combination. So I made myself give it a try. As expected, I hated it. It tasted like cardboard, not to mention the olives. Nevertheless, I forced myself to continue eating the same entrée of tomatoes, cumbers, and olives every morning. About two months into it, I began to notice something quite surprising: I was starting to look forward to what had become my standard breakfast. I even got to the point where I could not enjoy the tomatoes and cucumbers without my olives! Aside from benefiting my health, the experience taught me an invaluable lesson: that we learn to like whatever we eat on a regular basis. It's not a concept that I have heard much about, but it's the most powerful and practical advice I can give. So do some research and start eating whatever will optimize your health. Before long you will learn to like it as much as you like the way it makes you look and feel!

So there you have it. We started out by discussing the mental and emotional aspects of exercise and found that, in addition to its positive effects on the mind, exercise motivates us to eat healthfully--a habit that is fundamental to our mental, emotional, and physical well-being.

Principles of a healthy exercise routine

Never has there been such an explosion of exercise advice, routines, and devices. From aerobics and strength-training videos to in-home devices and total gyms, it seems that nearly every day there is a new workout routine or machine on the market. But with so many options and divergent opinions, one wonders, can they all be right?

In thinking about this, we must remember that the target audience for the fitness industry is primarily healthy young adults. Consequently, professional trainers and so-called "fitness gurus" can get away with a lot of mistakes in what they advertise and teach. A young body is a resilient one, and so the accuracy of what is being taught is seldom tested. But take someone who is older, injured, or severely debilitated, and the wisdom of what he or she is instructed to do will readily become apparent.

At the peak of my disability from a crippling injury that I sustained while exercising, I sought the help of some thirty health professionals that included physicians, chiropractors, physical therapists, fitness trainers, massage therapists, and just about every discipline in between. Being a physician, I sought and could afford the best. And humbled as I was by the gravity of my condition, I went into every assessment as open-minded and trusting as one could be. When after nearly four years of searching I still had not found anyone who was able to help me, I started to ask myself: had my problem been too complicated?

Had it become too far progressed? Or did none of the professionals I consulted really understand musculoskeletal pain and dysfunction? Well the answer to that question would have to wait until I found the answer to my problem, assuming I would ever find it.

By God's grace, I eventually did find the answer and with it the realization that none of the professionals I had consulted really understood the cause of musculoskeletal pain. And that is not my opinion alone. A few of them warned me that most of the people in the business did not have a comprehensive understanding of what they were teaching. Unfortunately, it turned out that the ones who warned me did not either.

So how could this be? How could so many professionals, many of them good-hearted and well-intended, be so lacking in their understanding and recommendations? Even more perplexing is that most of those recommendations were made with great confidence and assurance. The answer is that precious few people understand the complexities of muscle structure and function. Rather than working off new discoveries in basic science, most of the professionals who treat musculoskeletal disorders simply practice what they have been taught. Most of that teaching has been handed down from generations that predated modern discoveries about the neuromuscular system. Another barrier to education is that most of the individual discoveries about muscle were never integrated into a cohesive whole that could be applied to athletic training and the treatment of injuries. Instead, the information remained scattered throughout the pages of classic anatomy and physiology textbooks that have long since been shelved along with the valuable information they contain. Consequently, the quality of physical rehabilitation and fitness training has been limited to what professionals in the field have managed to learn from each other and their patients and clients.

Dr. Griner's research began to change all that. By the 1980s, he had begun to publish twenty-five years of painstaking work to integrate the hard science of muscle structure and function with age-old clinical observations to solve the mystery behind common musculoskeletal pain syndromes. The relevance of this to creating a healthy exercise routine is that one has to understand how muscles become sick before one can appreciate how to keep them well.

Recall that skeletal muscle is comprised of both slow and fast-twitch fibers. Slow-twitch fibers can burn both fats and proteins for energy, and they do that aerobically (using oxygen). The end products of their metabolism are carbon dioxide and water. Fast-twitch fibers are only able to burn carbohydrates, and they do that anaerobically (without oxygen). The first product of their metabolism is pyruvic acid. If there is enough oxygen in the muscle, most of the pyruvic acid can be metabolized aerobically by neighboring slow-twitch fibers. If there is not enough oxygen, up to half the pyruvic acid is converted to lactic acid. In either case, fast-twitch muscle is always producing some lactic acid.

Contrary to what one would think, our muscles are constantly working, even when we are completely relaxed or asleep. That's because continuous muscle tone is needed to prevent our joints from dislocating. Although our joints also have tough ligaments and capsules that hold them together, these inelastic structures are too loose (as they must be to allow freedom of movement) to secure the joint without the help of muscles and tendons. Now then, because our muscles are constantly working, they are constantly producing the end products of their metabolism: carbon dioxide and water by slow-twitch fibers, and lactic acid by fast-twitch fibers. So even at rest, our muscles are producing some lactic acid. However, blood and lymphatic circulation through muscle tissue is poor when muscles are at rest. Consequently, lactic acid accumulates in our muscles when we are inactive or asleep.

As previously discussed, accumulated lactic acid weakens the neurological signal that muscle spindles send to the brain. The cerebellum interprets this as a need to increase muscle tone, so it orders up more tension in the muscle. That is why we tend to be stiff in the morning or after we sit for a long time. Movement stimulates circulation through the muscles both by mechanical action and by the production of carbon dioxide, which is a vasodilator. The increased circulation carries away the accumulated lactic acid, and our muscles begin to loosen up. As they loosen, resistance to circulation progressively falls, which allows lactic acid to be carried away by the blood with increasing speed. It also increases oxygenation to the muscles, which helps reduce lactic acid production. That's why our muscles progressively loosen as we continue to move about. If we take it one step further and go for a leisurely walk, we will really cleanse and loosen the muscles.

But imagine what happens if we lead a sedentary lifestyle. You guessed it, the muscles will become increasingly burdened with lactic acid. This will continually drive up their resting tone until the rate of lactic acid production begins to exceed the rate at which the increasingly restricted circulation can remove it. The trapped lactic acid will create a self-perpetuating cycle of spasm while continuously poisoning the spindles. If this pattern goes on long enough or frequently enough, spindle feedback will remain distorted and continue even if all the trapped lactic acid occasionally gets flushed out. This is the condition that we have been referring to as hypertonic spasm. Although hypertonic spasm reduces the flexibility and functional capacity of muscle tissue, it usually goes unnoticed until it has progressed to the more superficial layers of the muscle, which are more sensate than the deeper layers. That is also the point where it involves enough of the muscle to irritate local nerves, impair routine functions, and result in injuries, such as when your neck locks up or you through out your back.

But there is more to the subject of muscle health than just preventing the accumulation of lactic acid in the muscles. Indirectly, lactic acid can be toxic to the blood vessels as well because when concentrated, it irritates the inside lining of the vessels, causing them to release histamine. Histamine drives the formation of atherosclerotic plaques by increasing cellular permeability to low-density lipoproteins, which accumulate in the cells and cause them to swell and harden. Histamine also drives the release of adrenaline, which raises blood pressure and causes the already narrowed arteries to spasm. Over time, these factors can come together to cause blood clots, strokes, and heart attacks. When you hear about the avid runner who died of a heart attack while running, the tragedy was more likely not an irony but rather the end result of chronic lactic acid toxicity. The long-term daily exposure to persistently high lactic acid levels caused by a continuous high-intensity exercise routine can gradually lead to atherosclerosis. This then sets the stage for a heart attack or stroke when the rising blood level of lactic acid and adrenalin cause an already narrowed coronary or cerebral artery to go into acute spasm.

The outpouring of adrenalin caused by high lactic acid levels can also precipitate panic attacks in susceptible individuals. The escalating fear experienced in a panic attack can then cause even more adrenaline to be released, which places such individuals at even greater risk from unhealthy exercise routines. Just ahead, we'll talk about healthier ways to exercise.

Another common example of the toxic effects of lactic acid is in the hemorrhoidal veins, which drain the anal sphincter muscle. The purpose of the anal sphincter is to prevent stool from leaking out of the bowel. In performing its function, the muscle is constantly active and dumping large quantities of lactic acid into the hemorrhoidal veins. Lactic acid causes the blood to thicken in the same way that it causes milk to thicken when produced by bacteria in the formation of yogurt. When the blood thickens in the hemorrhoidal veins, it can form clots that cause hemorrhoids to become thrombosed and painful. Another common site of venus clotting in association with lactic acid is deep in the calf and is known as a deep vein thrombosis or DVT.

So if we want to preserve our general health as well as our muscle health, we need to choose exercises and routines that will allow the circulatory system to wash lactic acid out of the muscles without driving up the blood levels in the process. The prototypical example of this is walking. A leisurely walk on level ground recruits both slow and fast-twitch fibers under a relatively mild work load, thus minimizing the production of lactic acid. When executed with the proper form, the slow pace also allows the veins in the calf muscles to completely refill between contractions, which improves circulation to the heart. The enhanced venus return to the heart does more than just give it a little more blood to pump. The heart's ability to generate force is partially dependent upon the degree to which it refills between contractions. Therefore, small increases in venous return can make large differences in the heart's ability to pump blood to all the muscles of the body, including those of the upper body even though they are not being used very much while walking. By optimizing circulation throughout the body, walking causes both the exercise-induced lactic acid and the previously accumulated lactic acid to be carried from the skeletal muscles to the heart and liver for clearance without very much raising the circulating concentration. The heart is capable of burning lactic acid for fuel, and the liver can recycle it into glucose for safe redistribution throughout the body.

To execute the most beneficial walking mechanics, plant your lead foot flat on the ground when you step forward, and push your body along by driving off the heal of your rear foot rather than off your toes. When performed properly, you should feel a slight stretch in the calf muscle of your rear leg as you take the step. As you take the next step, slightly lift your hip (rather than your thigh) and allow your leg to swing freely forward. Your foot should land flat, with your weight evenly distributed on your heels and toes rather than primarily on your heel. This puts the larger muscles to work, aiding circulation and minimizing the production of lactic acid. If you are not accustomed to walking this way, it might feel a little awkward at first, but it will soon become second nature. Even if you don't walk for exercise, you take thousands of steps each day, and getting into the habit of walking this way will be well worth the effort.

Running

In contrast to walking, running causes a build-up of lactic acid. Even at a relatively slow pace, running drives up the heart rate, thus giving the heart less time to refill between beats. It also gives the calf muscles, which are like accessory heart muscles when being used, less time to refill between contractions, thus reducing the amount of venous blood they pump back to the heart. Consequently, the amount of blood the heart pumps per beat during running is not as great as when walking, which translates to less circulation per lactic acid molecule produced. Running also preferentially recruits fast-twitch fibers because the force and speed with which the leg muscles must contract exceeds the capacity of slow-twitch fibers. This further increases the lactic acid burden. As the concentration of lactic acid rises in the blood, it irritates blood vessels and reduces the muscle-cleansing effect of the exercise because the recirculated blood is still polluted with lactic acid. Sensing the toxicity, the liver orders a rise in heart and respiratory rate in an effort to clear the excess acid. Thus, running exercises the heart and respiratory system more than walking, but it does so at the expense of flushing the accumulated lactic acid out of the muscles and protecting the vessel walls.

Those who enjoy running can get the best of both worlds if they continue to run at their preferred pace but walk for a bit every time they start feeling winded. Alternating between running and walking gives the heart and liver a chance to clear the excess lactic acid produced during the running phase of the routine. This will help ensure that the concentration of lactic acid in the blood remains in a safe range while still conditioning the cardiorespiratory system. It will also preserve the antidepressant effects of running. The same alternating pattern should be used for the other so-called "aerobic, fat-burning exercises," such as swimming, cycling, and elliptical machine. Those interested in losing weight should take note that none of these exercises is truly aerobic when performed continuously because of the preferential recruitment of fast-twitch fibers, which, as we have said, burn sugar rather than fat. So the good news is that by taking frequent breaks to slow down and catch your breath when running, you will be burning more fat in addition to exercising in a way that is both easier and healthier for you. Moreover, the muscles are worked more completely because of the more balanced recruitment of slow and fast-twitch fibers. Competitive athletes who feel that they must run hard continuously in order to build endurance are actually desensitizing their liver to circulating lactic acid. That's okay for a season, but those who continue this form of exercise on a long-term basis are placing themselves at ever-increasing risk of cardiovascular disease because of the pathologic vascular changes caused by concentrated lactic acid.

So to review what we have said, the correctly performed leisurely walk is the best way to detoxify skeletal muscle and keep it healthy and flexible. We can safely build strength and stamina through more vigorous exercises such as running, speed-swimming, and elliptical machine provided that we intermittently slow down to allow some of the excess lactic acid to be removed from the blood. Note that this alternating pattern is what naturally occurs in most competitive sports like baseball, basketball, football, soccer, hockey, and tennis. The alternating pattern also burns more fat and works the muscles more completely than if we push ourselves continuously.

Strength-training

The same principles of healthy exercise apply to strength-training. Recall that when round muscles contract, they squeeze their own blood vessels and lymphatics, choking off circulation. Hence, removal of the lactic acid that is accumulating in these muscles must await the return of circulation during the relaxation phase of the contraction. Also recall that both slow and fast-twitch fibers are recruited during slow movements but that slow-twitch fibers begin to drop out as the speed of movement increases, leaving the lactic acid-producing, fast-twitch fibers picking up an increasing share of the work. Consequently, slow movements during strength-training exercise more of the muscle and produce less lactic acid than fast movements. Slow movements also burn fat, not just glucose. But even slow movements can cause enough lactic acid build-up to poison the muscle spindles if the limited store of oxygen in the slow-twitch fibers becomes depleted. That's because a continuous supply of oxygen is needed by slow-twitch fibers to oxidize the pyruvate coming from fast-twitch fibers and prevent it from turning to lactic acid. The unwanted build up of lactic acid begins to occur after about six seconds of continuous muscle contraction.[8]

With the popular rush to look healthy and fit, an increasing number of men and women are looking to build shapely "cut" muscles. But because they are either unfamiliar with or fail to take into consideration the physiology of muscle, most trainers and their clients arc doing as much harm to their health as the overweight couch potato. Deceived by appearances, they teach and develop exercise routines that unknowingly drive more and more muscle into hypertonic spasm. Routines that involve prolonged muscle contractions such as holding a bridge pose and high-repetition pumping of weights routinely violate the six-second rule. That means they are causing lactic acid to accumulate in the muscles. The "pump" that these exercises are intended to achieve means that blood is pooling in the muscles as a result of the constricting effect that sustained muscle contraction has on the thin-walled vessels that drain the muscle of deoxygenated blood. The "burn" means that metabolic waste products, including lactic acid, are trapped in the muscle. Recall that once the muscle spindles become poisoned with lactic acid, the muscles will remain tense even at rest. While the excess tension functions to maintain the pump, it

57

also leads to hypertonic spasm. So that ripped, cut look that so many fitness buffs are after is anything but healthy; it's sickened muscles that are choking off their own blood supply. In addition to allowing lactic acid to accumulate in the tissue, the increased resistance to blood flow forces the heart to pump harder than normal. Over time, the heart can become hypertrophied and develop electrical disturbances that have been associated with an increased risk of cardiac sudden death.[9]

Spastic muscles also interrupt communication between the brain and vital organs by compressing and irritating nerves that pass through and between them. Nearly every organ and tissue of the body needs continuous neurological input to remain healthy and perform its normal functions; hypertonic muscle interrupts that lifeline. As an example, I had developed a spastic bladder and a rising PSA (prostate specific antigen) as the muscles in my back, hip, and leg continued to tighten over time. What helped me make the association between my bladder symptoms and my musculoskeletal problems was that my bladder would temporarily become more spastic after I would lift something heavy. I would also experience an increase in my foot symptoms, which made me suspect that whatever was irritating the nerves to my leg was also irritating the nerves to my bladder. Even more alarmingly, my PSA had more than doubled, jumping from 1.72 to 3.6 during the time that I was having sciatic nerve symptoms. The urologist was so concerned that he recommended a prostate biopsy to rule out prostate cancer. Though my doctors could not see how my rising PSA could be related to my nerve and muscle symptoms, the laboratory value gradually declined from 3.6 (at the height of my physical symptoms) to 2.6 (after three months of weekly KANON myotherapy), and finally to 1.4 (after an additional six months of therapy). Commensurate with the fall in PSA was a significant reduction in muscle spasticity and a gradual resolution of my bladder symptoms. Both the bladder and prostate are served by nerves of the pelvic plexus, and some of those nerves were likely being irritated by the iliopsoas (a large pelvic muscle) that had gone into spasm while doing a squatting exercise. So just as with improper aerobic training, improper strength-training can be as hazardous, and in some cases even more hazardous to one's health as not doing anything at all.

What makes this issue even more alarming is that once muscle goes into hypertonic spasm, it is trapped in a vicious cycle that is highly resistant to change. You can try stretching it, strengthening it, swimming it, pounding it, heating it, icing it, massaging it, electrocuting it; but none of these will free up whatever portion of the muscle has become hypertonic. I personally tried all of the above forms of treatment including daily swimming for three years without one bit of improvement. And there are no real warning signs that the tissue is becoming hypertonic. In fact, bodybuilders can look and feel as though they are doing themselves a lot of good, especially when they receive flattering complements about their physique, when in fact they could be setting themselves up for health problems later in life. For until hypertonic spasm incorporates most of the muscle, the only symptoms aside from looking and feeling good may be some stiffness or achiness that is assumed to be a natural consequence of training or aging. In some cases, the growing spasm might create a creaking sound called "crepitus," but that too can be misleading because it can sound as though it is coming from a joint. In reality, the creaking is the sound of tight, spastic muscles rubbing against one another and compressing the joints they are constantly stressing. So remember: whenever you strength-train incorrectly, you are unknowingly pushing your muscles into hypertonic spasm!

The healthier and more effective way to strength-train is to avoid holding any muscle or group of muscles in continuous contraction for more than six seconds. Muscles grow by being repeatedly stimulated; they need not be repeatedly poisoned through multiple rep exercises that cause lactic acid to accumulate. Sixteen sets of two reps provides the same growth stimulus as four sets of eight reps. Fewer reps also allows one to work up to a higher weight maximum, which has the potential of building even more muscle, if that is your goal. All movements should be performed slowly so as to work more of the muscle by stimulating both slow and fast-twitch fibers. Slow movements also burn fat, not just sugar, and produce less lactic acid in the process. Slow movements also help ensure good form, which, together with the recruitment of both slow and fast-twitch fibers, reduces the risk of injury. The correct application of these principles means doing multiple sets of two reps because with slow movements, you really can't do more than two reps without violating the six-second rule. Also, remember that muscles need at least thirty seconds of rest to detoxify and reoxygenate. The most efficient way to allow this is to circuit train opposing muscle groups; that way you can go directly from one exercise to another and still allow your muscles to rest without losing time standing around. If you do take a break, don't stand just stand there; walk around so that you use your calf muscles to optimize the circulation of deoxygenated blood back to your lungs. Always begin with light weights and work your way up as the blood supply to the muscles increases. Exercising this way builds more muscle in an easier, healthier, and safer way than doing continuous reps or holding muscles in isometric contraction. Finally, remember to breathe deeply and continuously while lifting both because it optimizes the availability of oxygen to the blood and because valsalva (breath-holding) while lifting can drive up blood pressure to the point of rupturing blood vessels. Every year a number of individuals, some of them young and otherwise healthy, are rushed to the hospital with a hemorrhagic stroke (ruptured blood vessel in the brain) due in part to breath-holding while pressing weights.

Even with the best of intentions, it can be difficult to adhere to the six-second rule unwaveringly. Anyone who works out on a regular basis knows that there are times when you feel so good and so strong that you just can't resist doing multiple repetitions. It's also a fact of life that we sometimes do things outside the gym that create hypertonic spasm, such as lifting and holding heavy items at work or, conversely, sitting at a desk for too long. The mere act of sleeping pushes our muscles in the direction of hypertonic spasm because blood is shunted away from muscles that are at rest for a long time.

As previously discussed, the brisk circulation that is stimulated by the simple act of walking cleanses the muscles of this toxic build-up. Hence, therapeutic walking should be part of every person's exercise routine. For those who primarily strength-train, walking should be done as a warm-up immediately before your routine and immediately afterward as a cool-down. If that's not possible, walking should be done on the off days, preferably in the morning, when the body is most burdened with toxins after lying in bed all night. The morning walk can really loosen you up in preparation for an active day. The need to walk applies to all of us regardless of our age, occupation, or level of fitness because all of us need to rid our muscles of toxic waste products on a regular basis if we want them to remain viable and strong as we age.

On a practical level regarding strength-training and exercise in general, any muscle that is heavily worked should be permitted to rest for at least seven days. Some experts say three days, but in my experience, seven to nine days is needed for full recovery. That's not to say that shorter rest periods will prevent strength and gains; it's just that the gains will not be as great because muscles need time to fully rebuild before they can fully benefit from being heavily worked again. The goal of proper strength-training is to stimulate the muscles enough to induce constructive (anabolic) changes with a minimum of destructive (catabolic) changes. Training too frequently offsets this balance and partially defeats it's purpose. Ample rest and moderation also prevents structural damage to tissues that need time to rebuild and strengthen to avoid being injured and possibly irreversibly damaged. Cardiorespiratory training should likewise be performed in moderation to prevent the body from becoming over-exhausted. Walking for exercise can be done six days a week, but more intensive cardiorespiratory training should be done no more than two to three times per week and for a duration of no more than twenty to thirty minutes per day. That might sound too minimalistic by today's standard, but let's remember that we are living in an era in which people are increasing impatient for results and losing sight of the fact that haste makes waste. Symptoms of over-training include the development of pain, fatigue, anxiety, irritability, and drowsiness. Overtraining also increases one's susceptibility to colds and flus because the body is too exhausted to fight off infectious pathogens. Dr. Kenneth Cooper, founder of the Cooper Institute for Aerobic Research and "the father of aerobic exercise" recanted his original assertions about cardiovascular fitness after watching a disproportionate number of his aerobic-enthusiast friends die of cancer and heart disease. After conducting tests to determine the maximum level of purely beneficial aerobic exercise, he found that anything in excess of twenty minutes per session has greatly diminishing returns and that if you double that amount, it negates all the initial benefits.[10] Of course, there will be individual differences and even personal differences as one ages or modifies his or her dietary habits and lifestyle, and so it behoves all of us to experiment and listen to our bodies. The key is to provide just enough stimulation to induce a training effect and then use proper nutrition, rest, and commitment to a regular exercise routine to accomplish the rest.

In an effort to prevent injury and promote longevity, we should build variety into our exercise routine. Instead of fixating on one form of exercise such as running, swimming, or weight-lifting, we should try to incorporate a balance of aerobic, cardiorespiratory, and strength-training. We should also add variety within each of these categories. The more we mix up the routine, the more versatile and resistant to injury we will become. If we are mindful to select at least one or two exercise activities that can be safely continued into old age, such as bicycling or golf, there may never be a need to stop exercising!

To recap what we have said, strength-training should be performed with slow movements and deep breathing. Muscles should not be held in contraction for more than six seconds without allowing them to completely relax for at least as much time. Muscles should also be given ample time to recover from an exercise session--a minimum of seven days for strength-training and forty-eight hours for cardiorespiratory training. Heavy lactic acid-producing exercises like weight-lifting, running, and swimming should be coupled with plenty of rest and some leisurely walking to help rid the muscles of lactic acid. Walking also adds variety to the exercise routine and is the only exercise that can be done every day without overly fatiguing the body.

Proper attention to the rules of exercise will safeguard you against overtraining and promote the development of plump muscles that are flexible and strong rather than tight muscles that are sculpted but inflexible and unhealthy. Contrary to what the popular "no pain no gain" mentality might tell us, the easier form of exercise, when executed properly, is healthier yet no less effective than dangerously pushing the body beyond its limit.

Proper warm-up

From what we have discussed so far, it stands to reason that a leisurely walk would be the ideal warm-up for more strenuous exercise because it would increase circulation and cleanse the muscles of lactic acid, thereby making them more relaxed, more flexible, and more resistant to injury. It is counterintuitive to think that a simple exercise like walking could "warm up" any muscles other than the legs, but because of the wholistic relationship between the muscles and the cardiovascular system, the simple act of walking actually detoxifies and prepares the upper body as well, though not to the extent that it does the lower body. Thus, walking should be combined with some gentle loosening of the upper body prior to engaging in strenuous physical activity.

Notice that I use the term "loosening" rather than "stretching." Many people attempt to loosen up by holding muscle groups in a stretched position, not realizing that this actually does more harm than good. Muscles are not designed to be stretched; they are designed to contract and relax. When muscles are held in a stretched position for more than a brief moment (the fraction-of-a-second that it takes to activate the stretch reflex), they reflexively contract in an effort to maintain joint integrity. Hence, traditional stretching actually makes muscles tighter and more prone to injury. Beyond that, repeated stretching can cause muscles and their tendons to become more fibrous, which is physiologically unhealthy. Muscles are not tight rubber bands or clumps of dough that will become more flexible through repeated stretching. Muscle is living tissue whose pliability is dependent upon its physiological state. So if we want to increase the health and flexibility of our muscles, we need to train the neuromuscular system to make the physiological adjustments that will permit our muscles to smoothly move through a greater range of motion. To accomplish this, we need to move through the intended range of motion without stimulating the stretch reflex. That requires slow, gentle movements in which we approach the end of the range of motion without pressing into it. Once there, we immediately return to neutral position to avoid activating the stretch reflex. When done properly, the muscle will feel like it is releasing rather than forcibly stretching. As blood flow increases and the muscles warm up, range of motion will naturally increase. The proper warm-up for a baseball pitcher, for example, would be to gently rotate his or her arm through the intended range of motion and then continue to loosen up by

THE GOLDEN BOOK OF MUSCLE HEALTH AND RESTORATION

throwing each successive pitch a little harder. The proper warm up for a runner would be to walk for several minutes and then gradually transition through intermittent jogging into running.

I have heard many people say that when they stretch-and-hold, they are able to increase their range of motion. But if you stretch to the point that it feels like you are pulling against a tight rubber band, then you are stretching the tendon, not the muscle. As previously stated, muscles do not stretch; they contract and relax. The tension you create when you hold the stretch is repeatedly activating the stretch reflex, which works to make the muscle shorter and tighter rather than longer and looser. However, if the tendon stretches more than the muscle shortens, it creates the false impression that the muscle has lengthened. Tendons are semi-elastic extensions of muscles that attach to bones. Stretching them might increase your range of motion, but over time it can cause them to thicken, lose flexibility, and create painful bone spurs. Furthermore, because stretching the tendon does not reduce tension in the muscle, it does nothing to increase circulation and cleanse the muscle of lactic acid. In other words, it does not increase muscle flexibility. On the contrary, it reduces flexibility and increases the risk of injury. You will be pleasantly surprised that when you warm-up by simply walking and gently moving your arms and legs through the intended range of motion, your performance will improve and your risk of injury will be less because your muscles will be more supple and capable of greater range of motion than by the faulty method of stretch-and-hold.

+ + +

CHAPTER 8

NUTRITION

No discussion of muscle health would be complete without addressing nutrition. We are the products of what we eat, and with the exception of cardiac tissue, cartilage, and some parts of the nervous system, our bodies are completely rebuilt every two years. And what are they made of? Whatever we put into our bodies during that time!

The human body is over sixty percent water by weight. That makes water the most important component of our diet. A human being can live for months without food but only weeks without water. Virtually every organ and tissue of the body needs adequate hydration to carry out its normal functions.

For those of us fortunate enough to live in a developed country, the concern is not severe dehydration but chronic mild dehydration because it is a silent contributor to the premature development of disease. The human body is like a plant, and when we are not adequately hydrated, we begin to wilt inside. Circulation is reduced to every organ and tissue, resulting in reduced cellular nutrition, detoxification, and immune function. As time goes on, the kidneys develop stones, the intestines develop diverticuli, and the muscles become hypertonic. These are just a few of the wide-ranging consequences of chronic mild dehydration. Most of the more familiar symptoms of dehydration, such as dry mouth, headache, and dizziness, do not occur unless dehydration is more severe. Consequently, we can live in a chronic state of mild dehydration without knowing it, which is as detrimental to our health as it is silent.

The biggest barrier to maintaining adequate hydration is that we often misinterpret a need for water as a need for food. This drives up appetite and we eat when all our body really needs is water. The confusion is not surprising given that most of the foods we eat have a high water content, not to mention that food intake is usually accompanied by fluid intake. That means the body usually gets water even if all it learns to ask for is food. Consequently, it has little impetus to maintain a distinct thirst signal for mild to moderate dehydration. Only when the body becomes severely dehydrated does it need to ask specifically for water...and it does. But the relative lack of a distinct warning signal for mild to moderate dehydration leaves us with the challenge of staying well-hydrated without eating more than our body really needs.

That is why I recommend drinking a glass of water at the first sign of hunger. If the hunger either persists or returns after five or ten minutes, then you know your body is needing food. If you then eat, the test-glass of water will pave the way for digestion without diluting the enzymatic activity that is stimulated by food intake. Another good habit is to drink a second glass of water about an hour after eating. This will keep food moving through the intestinal tract and help ensure that you don't start feeling hungry again until your body really needs another meal. Bear in mind that there is little advantage to drinking larger quantities of water all at once because the body rapidly excretes the excess. Under normal circumstances, all that is needed is about half a glass every two to three hours. To the extent that you keep your urine clear or colorless, you will know that you are doing a good job of staying well-hydrated.

By now you can appreciate the importance of water to muscle health understanding that water is needed in the blood to flush lactic acid out of the muscles and keep them plump, flexible, and strong. But like every other tissue of the body, muscles also need building blocks, especially if you are an athlete or are trying to build muscle through strength-training.

As discussed in the last chapter, exercise breaks down the body. The transient increase in muscle size and strength that occurs during a workout is merely the tissue heating up and filling with blood. The recovery phase is where the actual gains are made. So when it comes to muscle-building, what we do between workouts is even more important than what we do during workouts. Any experienced athlete knows that progress at building muscle is ten percent exercise and ninety percent diet. I would like to add that it is not only what we eat but how much we eat and when we eat it that is important. So we should also pay special attention to the timing and size of our meals.

Tests have shown that the physiologic sensation of hunger coincides with the disappearance of nutrients from the small intestine. That means that by the time the average person begins to feel hungry, the nutrient level in the blood is already starting to fall, and the body is beginning to feed on itself. The body looks to the liver cells for sugar, the fat cells for fat, and the muscle cells for protein. The longer we delay eating, the more muscle the body will break down to satisfy its protein needs. That's where the timing of meals becomes important.

The best way to ensure steady gains in strength and fitness is to provide the body with a steady stream of nutrients. To do this we need to eat soon enough after our last meal that we give the stomach time to digest and present what we have eaten to the duodenum (the first part of the small intestine) just as the last remains of the previous meal are being absorbed into the blood. It means we have to eat just before we begin to feel hungry. With practice and proper meal-planning, we can learn to achieve a seamless transition from meal to meal that has several important advantages. First, it provides the steady stream of nutrients that the body needs for daily activities and tissue repair. Second, it naturally reduces portion size because we are eating before we feel like eating. Third, it prevents the preprandial rise in insulin that is stimulated by thoughts of food as we begin to feel hungry. Insulin is a pancreatic hormone that directs the body to turn whatever we eat into fat and store it in our fat cells. That includes protein and carbohydrates. By eating before we begin to feel hungry, the insulin level remains lower, particularly if the meal is free of refined sugar. The lower the insulin level the more the body remains in fat-burning mode as opposed to fat-storing mode. More of the protein we eat will go to building muscle, and more of the carbs and fats will be converted to energy. In fact, if the meal is small enough, the body will not only turn it into energy, but it will burn some of the stored fat as well. The energy produced will leave us finishing our meals feeling more like exercising than laying down on the couch. So by simply eating small amounts just before you begin to feel hungry you will build more muscle, burn more fat, and feel more like working out. Imagine what a difference that will make in your physique! The mistake that most people make in their efforts to lose weight and get in shape is that they deprive themselves of food, which, as you can now see, causes muscle wasting, robs them of energy, and stimulates fat production.

A while back I had an experience that clearly illustrates the difference that the proper timing of meals can make. I had visited Israel on a tour of the Holy Land, and for ten days we spent most of each day walking through the desert in the hot sun without anything to eat between breakfast and dinner. Knowing that we would be going without lunch, I ate a whopping breakfast, and as hungry as I was by dinnertime, I ate an equally large dinner. In spite of the enormous size of my breakfast each morning, I spent at least four hours a day hungry because we never ate lunch. Now compare that to the standard way I had been eating prior to the trip, which consisted of the same kinds of foods but in much smaller quantities and always consumed just before I started to feel hungry. Also, I had been sitting most of the day in contrast to all the walking I did on the tour. When I returned from the trip, I was shocked to find that I had gained ten pounds! The experience was powerful proof that diet has a greater influence on our bodies than exercise. The experience also taught me that effective dieting should not leave you feeling like you are in the dessert; it just requires a careful timing of meals, and you won't even need to exercise to lose weight!

Yet in our high-pressured, fast-paced society, most persons do not take time to eat until they are really hungry. I've met some people who say they skip breakfast altogether, and others who say they skip both breakfast and lunch! These habits shut down metabolism for much of the day, leaving them in fat-building mode up to the time they eat their big evening meal, which, of course, the body converts to fat. No wonder they can't lose weight! And if they exercise regularly, it creates another problem: slow gains in the gym. They break down the body by exercising, and break it down even more by skipping meals. Unaware

68

of how much their eating habits are holding them back, many of them compound the problem by stepping up their exercise routine. Of course, that sets them back even further by further taxing a starved body. It's not surprising that some of them become so discouraged that they stop exercising altogether.

The good news is that establishing an effective routine is not that difficult; it just requires a little meal-planning and self-discipline. Any number of arrangements can be made, but the one I like best is to pack food from home and eat small amounts just before I begin to feel hungry. Of course, the perfect timing involves a little guess work at first, but before long you will become so good at it that you will frequently find yourself beginning to feel hungry just after you start eating. When that happens, you know you are getting fresh nutrients to the duodenum just as the last remains of what you had previously eaten are being absorbed. Eventually, maintaining this seamless transition from meal to meal will become second nature, and you will find yourself doing it on a regular basis without even thinking about it!

Last but by no means least, we must keep in mind that what we eat is even more important than when we eat it. There are two reasons for this. First, recall that we must avoid refined sugars in order to keep insulin levels low. Second, there is a difference between being lean and being healthy.

When it comes to physical health, there is no substitute for fresh fruits and vegetables. Of course, these high-carbohydrate foods should be combined with protein-rich foods, but the key word is *combined*. In his book The Zone Diet, Dr. Barry Sears presents elegant nutritional experiments that were performed on world class athletes to determine the optimal diet for health and fitness.*11* Because his study participants were highly disciplined and had established performance records, the effects of diet could be measured quantitatively. The results showed conclusively that the best diet for peak performance is not the high-protein diet, it's not the high-carbohydrate diet, it's not the high-fat diet; it's simply the balanced diet. That really should come as no surprise because like any building project, building up the body necessitates that the needed supplies be readily available at all times. That being said, we should try to include a healthy source of each of the three food groups in every meal. Healthy means foods that are low in saturated fats and contain the vitamins, minerals, and enzymes that allow the body to make the best use of the building blocks we give it. Some healthy sources of protein include fish, eggs, beans, yogurt, and nuts; healthy sources of carbohydrate include fruits, vegetables, and whole grains; and healthy sources of fat include avocados, fish, coconuts, olives, and nuts (with the exception of peanuts). Some foods, such as yogurt, nuts, and avocados, supply all three building blocks and, therefore, make ideal snacks.

Yogurt has the added advantage of supplying the friendly bacteria that boost immunity and aid digestion. Both our immune system and our digestive system are highly dependent upon the trillions of bacteria that colonize our intestinal tracts. Probiotic supplements are helpful, but even the best preparations fall short of supplying the wide variety of bacterial species that occupy the healthy bowel. Hence, they do not completely substitute for eating yogurt and other fermented foods containing live bacterial cultures on a regular basis. Unfortunately, all store-bought dairy products, including yogurt, are likely to be contaminated with Salmonella and Shigella. That's one of the little known reasons why milk causes gas and bloating for many people. What is commonly assumed to be lactose intolerance is frequently an age-related failure of stomach acids to kill pathogenic bacteria that get into processed milk despite pasteurization. Although small numbers of these pathogens usually cause little more than gas and temporary intestinal discomfort, they can be the source of "flu" outbreaks in the community, and repeated exposure can lead to more serious health problems down the road. To avoid this, simply boil all store-bought milk for ten seconds before drinking, and make your own yogurt. It's healthier, better-tasting, and less expensive than buying it pre-made. You can make yogurt with a yogurt-maker, or you can use the following age-old recipe.

Simply bring a half gallon or more of whole milk plus one pint of heavy whipping cream to a rising boil. Then shut the stove and allow the milk to cool to approximately 105° F (lukewarm). The cooled milk must remain warm enough to support bacterial growth but not be so warm that it destroys the starter culture you will be adding to it. Next, thoroughly mix a quarter cup of the warm milk into a quarter cup of store-bought plain yogurt, and pour the solution (starter culture) back into the pot before the milk cools much further. Gently stir for a few moments and then pour the entire pot of milk into a bowl that has been placed on a blanket. Cover the bowl with a plate and wrap it up with the blanket. The reason for the blanket is to help contain the heat in the culture medium. As the bacteria multiply, they produce lactic acid, which causes the culture to thicken into yogurt. This normally takes about nine hours. Once the culture has thickened, the yogurt is done and should be refrigerated. If you refrigerate the yogurt shortly after it thickens, it will be less tart. The longer you leave it out, the more tart it will become because of the continued production of lactic acid. You should save about half a cup of the newly made yogurt as starter culture for your next batch of home-made yogurt. For the best tasting first batch of yogurt, I recommend Oberwies whole milk and Horizen organic heavy whipping cream with Fage Greek yogurt as the starter.

Although any store-bought starter yogurt probably contains some pathogenic microorganisms, the degree of contamination in the finished yogurt will be negligible because any bad bacteria in the large pot of milk were killed when you boiled it. As the re-cultured yogurt incubates, the growth of friendly bacteria increasingly outweighs that of any harmful bacteria. This phenomenon is repeated each time you save a small amount of home-made yogurt to inoculate your next batch, thus steadily increasing the purity of each batch you make.

Another dietary pearl is to harness the power of juicing. A glass of fresh carrot or leafy green juice taken immediately before a work-out is a great way to hydrate the body while at the same time giving yourself a dose of super-nutrition. Unlike tap or even filtered water, fruits and vegetables contain organically purified water. You can't do much better than that. In addition, carrots contain virtually every nutrient the body needs, and leafy greens contain chlorophyll, which is stored solar energy that is released in the body when the juice is consumed. By letting the juicer do the work of digestion, all the nutrition in this rocket fuel becomes available for exercise. I'll never forget the first few times I juiced some carrots. The first time, I had been ready for an afternoon nap, but after drinking the carrot juice, three hours passed before I realized that I had continued to work right through my planned break. The next day, I had another glass of carrot juice, and about fifteen minutes later, I spontaneously dropped to the floor and started doing pushups. After that, I changed into a pair of shorts and went for a half-hour jog. Though I can't say that I experience such dramatic effects every time I juice, the energy boost can be amazing, and the nutritive value superb. It's important to consume these juices immediately because they rapidly oxidize, which destroys some of their beneficial effects. If you are interested in juicing, I recommend that you start by doing some on-line research. The information will help you select the proper juicer, and there are some potential pitfalls, such as developing kidney stones from consuming too many high-oxalate vegetables. So start out slow, and as with all things, practice moderation.

For those who have no interest or time for juicing, I would recommend a serving of fresh fruit combined with a proteinaceous food before a workout. There is no need to juice fruits because they are easily digested, and their sugar content can get you in the mood for exercise within just fifteen or twenty minutes. I have found grapes and an avocado to be a great pre-workout snack. In addition to all the health advantages they have over refined sugars, fruits have a lower glycemic index, which translates to a more even and sustained energy boost. An alternative to fruits is to have a snack that includes a teaspoon or two of honey. This is especially effective for those who do not normally eat sweets because their system has a heightened sensitivity to the sugar. However, I do not recommend eating the honey by itself; it should be combined with slower-digesting carbohydrates or healthy grains and a protein-rich food in order to maintain adequate blood sugar and the amino acids your muscles will need for repair. If the honey is locally-grown and consumed on a regular basis during the months leading up to allergy season, it can also help reduce or eliminate seasonal allergies because it contains some of the allergens that will help desensitize your immune system to those in your environment.

That brings us to the topic of powdered protein and other nutritional supplements. Although there is no doubt that whey and other protein formulations enhance muscle growth, they can eventually cause food allergies or even more severe health problems. It is far better and safer to carefully explore and combine natural foods because there is no way to improve upon what God has made. If there is one thing I have learned as a physician and scientist, it is that our understanding of the human body will never be comprehensive enough to make supplements that are completely safe. Anything unnatural carries the risk of stressing the body and throwing it out of balance in one direction or another. There are times when we have to take that risk, such as when treating an illness, but whenever there is a natural alternative, we would be wise to choose it even if it threatens to reduce the speed at which we race toward our objectives. Better to take a sure path than an uncertain one; better to arrive a little later than not at all.

There are several other important principles of a healthy diet, such as avoiding processed foods, opting for organically grown fruits and vegetables, and getting enough fiber, but that's getting beyond the scope of this book. For the purpose of our discussion, the secret to health and fitness boils down to meal planning and food selection in combination with a healthy exercise routine. You would be wise to establish the habit of preparing healthy snacks and eating them just before hunger strikes. The same applies to the consumption of water. We should not habitually make our bodies beg for what we know they need. Combining these dietary principles with a carefully designed exercise routine will help you get into the best shape of your life.

+ + +

About the Author

MICHAEL R. BINDER, M.D., is a gifted athlete who played baseball, basketball, football, and hockey at the competitive level before going to medical school and becoming a physician. At the age of forty, he had a thriving psychiatric practice and was physically in the best shape of his life, adhering to a zone diet and a rigorous exercise routine that combined swimming, running, and strength-training.

As he became increasingly involved in his work as a physician, the needs of his patients began to crowd out his own needs. Eventually, he became ill himself, suffering several attacks of kidney stones followed by a crippling back injury that created overwhelming emotional, physical, and spiritual distress. He would spend the next six years of his life trying to recover his health. In the process, he sought the help of over thirty healthcare professionals from a variety of disciplines, only to discover how little the "experts" really knew about his condition and how much pain and suffering others with similar injuries endure in their efforts to regain their health.

Through these trying years, Dr. Binder asked God to help him renew his strength and turn his suffering into a help to others by unveiling the mystery behind chronic musculoskeletal pain. This book is God's answer to his prayer.

References

1. Filler AG, Haynes J, Jordan SE, Prager J, Villablanca JP, Farahani K, McBride DQ, Tsuruda JS, Morisoli B, Batzdorf U, Johnson JP. *Sciatica of Nondisc Origin and Piriformis Syndrome: Diagnosis by Magnetic Resonance Neurography and Interventional Magnetic Resonance Imaging with Outcome Study of Resulting Treatment.* Journal of Neurosurgery - Spine 2005; Feb 2(2): 99-115.

2. Benson RT, Tavares SP, Marshall RW. *Conservatively Treated Massive Prolapsed Discs: a 7-year Follow-up.* Annals of the Royal College of Surgeons of England 2010; March 92(2): 147-153.

3. El Barzouhi A, Vleggeert-Lankamp CLAM, Lycklama à Nijeholt GJ, Van der Kallen BF, Van den Hout WB, Jacobs WCH, Koes BW, Peul WC. *Magnetic Resonance Imaging in Follow-up Assessment of Sciatica.* New England Journal of Medicine 2013; 368: 999-1007.

4. Moseley JB, Jr., Wray NP, Kuykendall D, et al. *Arthroscopic Treatment of Osteoarthritis of the Knee: a Prospective, Randomized, Placebo-controlled Trial. Results of a Pilot Study.* American Journal of Sports Medicine 1996; 24(1):28-34.

5. Burns JW, Loecker TH, Fischer JR Jr, Bauer DH. *Prevalence and Significance of Spinal Disc Abnormalities in an Asymptomatic Acceleration Subject Panel.* Aviation, Space, and Environmental Medicine 1996; 67: 849–853.

6. Crelin ES. *A Scientific Test of Chiropractic's Subluxation Theory. The First Experimental Study of the Basis of the Theory Demonstrates that it is Erroneous.* American Scientist 1973; September/October.

7. Johnson RM, Crelin ES, White AA 3rd, Panjabi MM, Southwick WO. *Some New Observations on the Functional Anatomy of the Lower Cervical Spine.* Clinical Orthopaedics and Related Research 1975; Sep (111): 192-200.

8. Griner T. *What's Really Wrong With You? A Revolutionary Look at How Muscles Affect Your Health.* Avery Publishing 1995.

9. Kang YJ. *Cardiac Hypertrophy: A Risk Factor for QT-Prolongation and Cardiac Sudden Death.* Toxicological Pathology 2006; 34(1): 58-66.

10. Cooper, KH. *Antioxidant Revolution.* T. Nelson Publishers 1994.

11. Sears B. *The Zone Diet.* Thorsons Publishers 1999.

Other Books by Michael R. Binder, M.D.

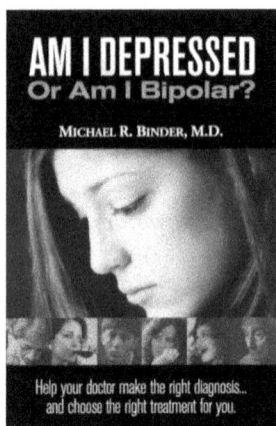

Am I Depressed Or Am I Bipolar?

This groundbreaking book will help you understand mood disorders from an anatomical, psychological, and spiritual perspective with an emphasis on making the distinction between classic depression and bipolar disorder. Drawing from years of clinical experience, research, and intensive study, board-certified psychiatrist Dr. Michael Binder unveils the anatomy of the mind and uses numerous case examples to familiarize you with the various forms that mood disorders can take. Throughout the book, he also discusses how they are properly diagnosed and treated.

Available at www.barnesandnoble.com and www.amazon.com

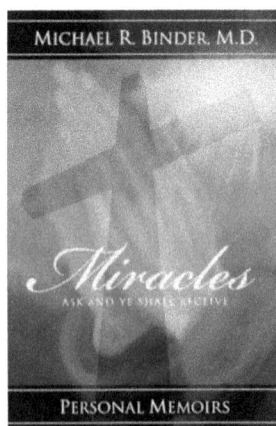

Miracles: Ask and Ye Shall Receive

Miracles is a book of personal memoirs that recounts the acts of God in the life of Dr. Michael Binder, a physician and scientist, who has witnessed the loving hand of God through faith time and again. Packed with more than one hundred miracles, this inspirational work describes the experiences of the doctor himself, which are presented with the historical accuracy and detail that one would expect from a clinical scientist. Those who believe in God will be strengthened by this book; those who are uncertain will be inspired; and those who do not believe will be challenged to take the leap of faith that opens the door to heaven on earth. Available at www.barnesandnoble.com and www.amazon.com

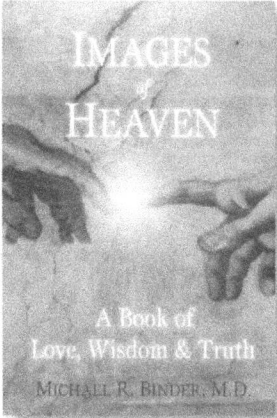

Images of Heaven: A Book of Love, Wisdom & Truth

This unique work is a study of the Holy Bible through the lens of science. Based on the most authentic complete Bible manuscripts in existence, Dr. Michael Binder combines his medical training and experience as a psychiatrist with the knowledge and insights of world-renown Bible scholar Dr. George M. Lamsa to help you understand the entire Bible, from the book of Genesis to the book of Revelation, in the language of our modern culture and times.

Images of Heaven is available only through The Binder Foundation. To learn more or to place an order, go to www.binderfoundation.com.

www.ingramcontent.com/pod-product-compliance
Lightning Source LLC
Chambersburg PA
CBHW052102270326
41931CB00012B/2860